Learning from Occupational Therapy in Latin America

of related interest

Occupational Identity
Journeys of Minoritized Occupational Therapists Across Race, Religion, and Culture
Alaa Abou-Arab and Erica V. Herrera with the Coalition of Occupational Therapy Advocates for Diversity
ISBN 978 1 83997 820 3
eISBN 978 1 83997 821 0

Antiracist Occupational Therapy
Unsettling the Status Quo
Edited by Musharrat J. Ahmed-Landeryou
Foreword by Professor Elelwani Ramugondo
ISBN 978 1 83997 574 5
eISBN 978 1 83997 575 2

Occupational Therapy Disruptors
What Global OT Practice Can Teach Us About Innovation, Culture, and Community
Sheela Roy Ivlev
Foreword by Juman Simaan
ISBN 978 1 83997 665 0
eISBN 978 1 83997 666 7

The Core Concepts of Occupational Therapy
A Dynamic Framework for Practice
Jennifer Creek
Foreword by Anne Lawson-Porter
ISBN 978 1 84905 007 4
eISBN 978 0 85700 362 1

The Essential Guide for Newly Qualified Occupational Therapists
Transition to Practice
Edited by Ruth Parker and Julia Badger
ISBN 978 1 78592 268 8
eISBN 978 1 78450 558 5

Learning from Occupational Therapy in Latin America

TRANSFORMATIVE APPROACHES FOR SOCIAL JUSTICE AND INCLUSIVE PRACTICE

Pamela Talero Cabrejo,
Vagner Dos Santos,
and **Nicholas Pollard**

FOREWORD BY ROSHAN GALVAAN

Jessica Kingsley Publishers
London and Philadelphia

First published in Great Britain in 2025 by Jessica Kingsley Publishers
An imprint of John Murray Press

2

A CIP catalogue record for this title is available from the British Library and the Library of Congress

ISBN 978 1 83997 389 5
eISBN 978 1 83997 390 1

Printed and bound in the United States by Integrated Books International

Jessica Kingsley Publishers' policy is to use papers that are natural, renewable and recyclable products and made from wood grown in sustainable forests. The logging and manufacturing processes are expected to conform to the environmental regulations of the country of origin.

Jessica Kingsley Publishers
Carmelite House
50 Victoria Embankment
London EC4Y 0DZ

www.jkp.com

John Murray Press
Part of Hodder & Stoughton Ltd
An Hachette Company

The authorised representative in the EEA is Hachette Ireland,
8 Castlecourt Centre, Dublin 15, D15 XTP3, Ireland (email: info@hbgi.ie)

To our families, students, and colleagues, and to the hundreds of voices across Latin America and beyond, whose everyday actions, reflections, and resistance give life and purpose to this work. May this book honor your wisdom, struggles, and dreams, and contribute meaningfully to the ongoing effort to democratize knowledge, so it may flow freely across borders, languages, and histories, in pursuit of a more just and inclusive world.

Contents

Part 3: Territories

Part 4: Arenas

The Editors

Pamela Talero Cabrejo, OTD, BSOT(Col), CPAM, COT
Assistant Professor, Post-Professional Occupational Therapy Program
Thomas Jefferson University, Philadelphia, PA, USA
Pamela.Talero@jefferson.edu

Vagner Dos Santos, Ph.D., MSc, BappSc, OT
Senior Lecturer in Occupational Therapy
School of Allied Health, Exercise and Sports Sciences
Charles Sturt University, Australia
vdossantos@csu.edu.au

Nicholas Pollard, Ph.D., MSc, BA (Hons), DipCOT
Senior Lecturer in Occupational Therapy
Department of Allied Health Professions
Sheffield Hallam University, Sheffield, UK
N.Pollard@shu.ac.uk

The Contributors

Albino, Andrea F. is an Occupational Therapist and a member of the Argentinean Association of Occupational Therapists (AATO). She is also Faculty at the University of Buenos Aires, National University of San Martín, and National University of Lanús. afalbino@hotmail.com

Akemi Takeiti, Beatriz is an Occupational Therapist with a Ph.D. in psychology and Faculty at the Federal University of Rio de Janeiro, Brazil. biatakeiti@medicina.ufrj.br

Alzamora Muñoz, Consuelo Cristina is an Occupational Therapist at the Tous Ensemble Foundation, Les Cayes, Haiti. consuelo.am@gmail.com

Becerra Becerra, Aida del Pilar is an Occupational Therapist and Master in Disability and Social Inclusion. She is the Agua Maestra collective coordinator and contractor at the Colombian Institute of Family Welfare, Bogotá, Colombia. adbecerrab@unal.edu.co

Bianchi, Pamela Cristina is an Occupational Therapist with a Ph.D. in Occupational Therapy. She is Faculty at the Federal University of São Paulo, Santos, Brazil. pamela.bianchi@unifesp.br

Castro de Jong, Daniela, Ph.D., MA, OT(Reg), GCTE, FHEA is a Nexus Fellow (Senior Lecturer) at the School of Health Sciences, UNSW Sydney, Australia. d.castro_de_jong@unsw.edu.au

Chambilla Tarqui, Lina Carla holds a Bachelor's in Educational Administration from the Catholic University of Bolivia and a Bachelor's in Occupational Therapy from the Universidad Mayor de San Andrés in Bolivia. carla.chambilla@gmail.com

Corrêa de Macedo, Maria Daniela, Ph.D. (Psychology) is a Professor at the Federal University of Rio de Janeiro, Brazil. mariadaniela@medicina.ufrj.br

Cristancho, Livet Rocío is a Colombian Occupational Therapist with a Master's in Public Health, a Ph.D. student in Occupational Therapy at the Universidade Federal de Sao Carlos, Brazil, and an assistant editor at *Revista Ocupación Humana*, Colombia. livetcristancho@gmail.com

Cruz Perdomo, Jaqueline is a Professor at the University of Valle, Colombia. She holds a Doctorate in Education from the University of Valle. jaqueline.cruz@correounivalle.edu.co

Daneri, Sara M. is an Occupational Therapist and a member of the Argentinean Association of Occupational Therapists (AATO) and the Latin American Confederation of Occupational Therapists (CLATO). She is Faculty at the Catholic University of La Plata, Bahía Blanca branch, and Gastón Dachary University. saramdaneri@gmail.com

Falleiros Braga, Iara is an Occupational Therapist, a Master and Doctor of Science, and a Professor at the Federal University of Paraíba, João Pessoa, Paraíba, Brazil. iarafalleiros@gmail.com

Farias, Lisette, Ph.D., MScOT, OT(Reg.) is an Assistant Professor in the Division of Occupational Therapy, Department of Neurobiology, Care Sciences and Society, Karolinska Institutet (Sweden). lisette.farias.vera@ki.se

Fernández Orellana, María Cristina is an Occupational Therapist, MA in Health Sciences Education, Ph.D. Student in Public Policy, and Academic at the School of Occupational Therapy, Faculty of Medicine and Health Sciences, Universidad Mayor, Santiago, Chile. maria.fernandez@umayor.cl

Herrera Bonilla, Alicia is an Occupational Therapist at Central Hospital of the Peruvian Air Force, with a Master's from the Universidad Nacional Mayor de San Marcos. aherrerab@unmsm.edu.pe

Lapierre, Michelle, MPH, OT is a Ph.D. Assistant Professor in the Department of Rehabilitation Sciences, Universidad de La Frontera (Chile). michelle.lapierre@ufrontera.cl

Llerena, Bryan Esteban is an Occupational Therapist with a Master's in Social and Community Intervention in Quito, Ecuador. bestebanllerena@gmail.com

Lopes Correia, Ricardo is an Occupational Therapist with a Ph.D. in Health Sciences. He is in the Faculty of Medicine at the Federal University of Rio de Janeiro, Brazil. ricardo@medicina.ufrj.br

López Díaz, Yenny Patricia is an Occupational Therapist and holds a Master's in Lifelong Learning in Multicultural Contexts and a Doctorate in Education. She is an Education Technician for Global Citizenship, Zaragoza, Spain. yennylopezdiaz@gmail.com

Marques, Ana, Ph.D., MSc (Sociology) is an Occupational Therapist (Reg.) and Lecturer in many occupational therapy training institutes in France, Coordinator of the program Prévention et Promotion de la Santé Mentale par des Activités Collectivisantes sur les Territoires (PRACTS), and an Associate Researcher at Projeto Metuia, Federal University of Sao Carlos (Brazil). a.marques@epsve.fr

Mondaca, Margarita, Ph.D., MSc(OT), OT(Reg.) is Assistant Professor in the Division of Occupational Therapy, Department of Community Medicine and Rehabilitation, Umeå University (Sweden), and affiliated to the Division of Occupational Therapy, Department of Neurobiology, Care Sciences and Society, Karolinska Institutet (Sweden). margarita.mondaca@ki.se

Monzeli, Gustavo Artur is an Occupational Therapist with a Ph.D. in occupational therapy. He is also Faculty at the Federal University of Paraíba, João Pessoa, Brazil. gustavo.monzeli@gmail.com

Morrison, Rodolfo is an Occupational Therapist with a Ph.D. in Logic and Philosophy of Science from Universidad de Las Américas (Chile), and Director and Associate Professor of the Department of Occupational Therapy and Occupational Science at the University of Chile (Chile). morrison.rodolfo@gmail.com

Navarrete Rodríguez, Gabriela Elizabeth, OT, MSc is an occupational therapist at Fundación Hermano Miguel. navarrete.gabriela.to@gmail.com

Nunes Farias, Magno is Professor at the University of Brasilia. He holds a Doctorate in Education from the Federal University of São Carlos, Brasilia, Brazil. magno.farias@unb.br

Painemal Morales, Lincoyan is an Occupational Therapist from the University of Bolivariana, Chile, and a current Professor at Santo Tomás University. lincoyan.painemal@gmail.com

Pedernera, María, OT, MSc is an Occupational Therapist and a member of the Paraguayan Association of Occupational Therapists. marisupedernerag@gmail.com

Pérez, Orlando Enrique is an Occupational Therapist at the Instituto Panameño de Habilitación, Universidad Especializada de las Américas, and a member of the Association of Occupational Therapists of Panama (ATOP). porlandoenrique@gmail.com

Ramírez Osorio, Diana Milena is an Occupational Therapist and Specialist in Public Health Management. She holds a Master's in Social Policy and Community Mediation. dmramirezo@unal.edu.co

Ramírez Ramírez, Roger Rodolfo is an Occupational Therapist and Faculty at the Universidad Católica de Temuco, Chile. rramirez@uct.cl

Rey, Andrés is an Occupational Therapist and Faculty at the University School of Medical Technology, Faculty of Medicine, University of the Republic in Uruguay. reydocencia@gmail.com

Riquelme Echeverría, Viviana is an Occupational Therapist at the University of Chile, a Psychologist, and holds a Master's in Occupational Therapy from Universidad Andrés Bello. She is an Academic in the Department of Occupational Therapy and Occupational Science at the University of Chile. vriquelme@uchile.cl

Rocha Santos, Francia Elena is an Occupational Therapist in Colombia. She is an Educator and Psychosocial Professional at the National University of Colombia. ferochas@unal.edu.co

Rodríguez Uzcátegui, Elizabeth, OT, PT is Faculty at the University College of Rehabilitation "May Hamilton" in Venezuela and is a member of the Venezuelan Federation of Occupational Therapists (FVTO). elizarodriguez15@gmail.com

Samacá Pulido, Julián is a Ph.D. Student in Philosophy at Universidade Federal do Espírito Santo, Brazil, with an Interdisciplinary Master's in Social Intervention from Alberto Hurtado University, Chile, and is a Colombian Occupational Therapist from the National University of Colombia. juliansto@gmail.com

Silva, Carla Regina is an Occupational Therapist, Ph.D. in Education, and Faculty at the Federal University of São Carlos, Brazil. carlars@ufscar.br

Valdelomar Marín, Erick is an Occupational Therapist, Specialist in Dementia Syndromes, and Specialist in Risk and Harm Reduction. He is the Director of the School of Occupational Therapy of the University of Santa Paula, Costa Rica. evaldelomar@uspsantapaula.com

Valderrama Nuñez, Cristian is Faculty at the Occupational Therapy School, Faculty of Health, Universidad Santo Tomás, Chile. He holds a Master's in Occupational Therapy from Andres Bello University, Chile. cristianvalderramanu@santotomas.cl

Foreword

A TAPESTRY OF DISSENT AND RADICAL HOPE

Many readers intimately familiar with occupational therapy will recognize the tensions with how it is conceptualized and practiced with an individualistic, biomedical orientation. The authors of the various chapters in this book offer compelling perspectives that move beyond describing these tensions, predominantly influenced by the Global North, critically examining the forces impacting the profession. This examination occurs from the position of Abya Yala (Latin America), appreciating the perspective of cosmovision and ancestral, Indigenous, and local knowledge. At a time of global discord, when the vigorous clamor for power, control, and dominance abounds, this book presents a beacon for how occupational therapy can learn and expand knowledge from the voices of Abya Yala and the broader Global South, voices historically silenced and overshadowed by the Anglophone. The authors persuasively argue for a more inclusive occupational therapy where the Global North and South learn reciprocally and respectfully from each other, dismantling longstanding hierarchies and exclusions.

A diverse tapestry of activist scholars advances the use of praxis embedded in critical theories, challenging us to question the foundations upon which our discipline and profession stand. They demonstrate the intersections of colonization, racism, patriarchy, neoliberalism, and epistemicide that have shaped occupational therapy. By incisively probing these intersections, the book critiques how dominance is re-inscribed in all facets of occupational therapy, including professional identities, to uphold unjust power dynamics and inequalities. Offering historical analyses, autobiographical reflections, case vignettes, and theoretical insights, the authors invite us into dialogue to re-sculpt our epistemological foundations and to think from the margins. These authors courageously reveal themselves, their experiences, and their thinking for the benefit of the profession as a collective. This illustrates how thinking with and from the margins of Indigenous, collective, critical, feminist, decolonial, anti-racist, and similar perspectives enables us, as a profession, to go alongside and beyond, to expand community collaboration, ancestral wisdom, social solidarity, and transformative justice. It delinks (Mignolo, 2007) occupational therapy from forms of knowledge that legitimize hegemony, amplifying possibilities for generative disruption.

Generative disruption (Galvaan, 2021) is demonstrated epistemically and pragmatically across the chapters, showing how to enact occupational therapy's social, political, and ethical responsibilities. The authors connect the interplay between the Global South's historical, sociopolitical, economic, and cultural struggles with processes and forms of deep spiritual and natural relations from Abya Yala and with Afrika. Significantly, this work is more than just a critique. It presents an active and hopeful contribution that deepens and extends critically conscious occupational therapy. It enables us to contribute to generative disruption by contemplating, deliberating, and subversively transgressing in ways that will build critical consciousness and political agency.

The authors write with unmistakable authenticity, offering an inspiring reimagining of hope. This hope transcends a mere utopian vision of the future. By weaving language, methods, and concepts laden with socially transformative potential, we are encouraged to engage in critical exchange with their ideas. They invite the occupational therapy community and beyond to challenge homogenizing and oppressive systems. Their approach is rooted in and responsive to the challenges we face locally and globally. Importantly, they do not provide a fixed blueprint or practice model. The essence of radical hope lies in the potential for different future possibilities that question what is taken for granted and make space for the silenced voices and languaging of the Global South. This book is a gift and a challenge for educators, students, practitioners, and researchers unaware, unsure, or afraid of doing differently. It gifts us profound insights and new vocabularies to engage meaningfully with the complex realities shaping global understandings of human occupation. To date, much of this has been inaccessible to the Anglosphere.

The need for this provocative text is especially urgent as the world continuously confronts the structures of power that emerged as a consequence of colonialism and that continue to shape political, social, cultural, economic, and epistemic relations. We must respond to this book's collective call to dissent: to honor the lived experiences, identities, wisdom, and needs of all communities, especially those historically marginalized and silenced.

May this text agitate meaningful conversations, inspire transformative praxis, and contribute significantly to re-imagining a more socially just and inclusive occupational therapy worldwide. As an elegantly packaged tapestry of dissent, it challenges us to do all we can to take action, to become critically reflexive and politically engaged.

With gratitude,
Roshan Galvaan, Professor, University of Cape Town, South Africa

References

Galvaan, R. (2021). Generative disruption through occupational science: Enacting possibilities for deep human connection. *Journal of Occupational Science, 28*(1), 6–18. https://doi.org/10.1080/14427591.2020.1818276

Mignolo, W. (2007). Delinking: The rhetoric of modernity, the logic of coloniality and the grammar of de-coloniality. *Cultural Studies, 21*(2–3), 449–514.

Introduction

While occupational therapy originated in North America and Europe in the early 20th century, its evolution outside these regions, particularly Latin America, remains significantly underrepresented in anglophone literature. This book, the first comprehensive English-language exploration of Latin American occupational therapy, seeks to fill this gap, presenting the region's culturally grounded approaches and critical discourses that offer essential perspectives on the profession. These contributions reflect a rich diversity predating the arrival of colonial occupational therapists in the 1950s and provide profound insights into the social, historical, and environmental realities shaping Latin American practice. Despite previous individual contributions to anglophone journals, a cohesive narrative of Latin American occupational therapy's evolution has been lacking. This absence prompted the editors and over 30 contributors to undertake this extensive project. It bridges languages and worldviews, creating essential dialogues for a more inclusive and globally connected profession.

For more than 65 years, Latin American occupational therapists have advanced transformative theoretical insights, influenced public policy, and developed educational, research, and practice frameworks. Yet these developments have remained largely unknown to anglophone audiences. This book expands the influence of Latin American perspectives, promoting networks, conceptual models, and representations that reflect the region's complex occupational therapy landscape. By fostering a greater understanding of these approaches, this work aims to contribute to global health practices and bridge the historical gaps between occupational therapy and occupational science, creating pathways for a more inclusive, worldwide dialogue.

Over the decades, Latin American occupational therapy has developed a robust discourse grounded in indigenous knowledge, postcolonial narratives, grassroots resistance, and innovative frameworks. While concepts such as social occupational therapy are now recognized in the Global North, colonial legacies and epistemic imbalances—forces that have suppressed non-Western ways of knowing—still mean that Latin American professionals may be more familiar with the histories of colonizing nations than their own. This book offers a compelling counterpoint, a cohesive exploration of Latin American occupational therapy's evolution that directly voices the intellectual and practical contributions of those who live and work within these diverse communities.

For those unfamiliar with Latin America, the region may seem exotic and enigmatic, often portrayed in dominant discourse as a place of contrast and complexity. However, this book seeks to demystify the region and presents *Abya Yala*—the Indigenous term transcending colonial boundaries and reflecting a deeply interconnected Latin America (see Chapters 2 and 3). Through this lens, readers are invited to let go of strict categories and reflect on human occupations with a fresh perspective, seeing occupational therapy in Latin America as an evolving journey of reflexivity, resistance, praxis, and community. Against a backdrop of colonial, postcolonial, and neocolonial struggles, this work offers a narrative and reflective journey through Latin American occupational therapy. It encourages us to connect from our current spaces and times to dialogue, empathize with universal human experiences, and consider what it means to coexist in a fragile world.

The book is the product of extended collaboration and exchange. Initially, the editors—Nick Pollard, a British occupational therapist with decades of dialogue and travel within Latin America; Vagner Dos Santos, a Brazilian occupational therapist based in Australia; and Pamela Talero Cabrejo, a Colombian occupational therapist residing in the United States—began their work individually but soon saw the potential for a collective project. Nick's interest in Latin American occupational therapy began early, sparked by books such as *The Voyages of Christopher Columbus* (Waldman, 1964) and *Ferdinand Magellan* (Groh, 1966). This childhood fascination grew into a deep understanding of colonialism's destructive impact on the region. In his later encounters with Chilean refugees, and through the literature of Borges, García Márquez, Vargas Llosa, and Freire's *Pedagogy of the Oppressed* (1970), he began to recognize the vital importance of Latin American perspectives in global occupational therapy discourse. Vagner has collaborated extensively with South American colleagues, co-editing two *Contemporary Questions and Practices of Occupational Therapy* editions in South America (Dos Santos & Gallassi, 2014; Dos Santos, Muñoz, & Farias, 2022). Pamela has worked in community-based participatory approaches that emphasize addressing social inequities. Through their collaborations across the region, each editor has contributed to shaping a project that aspires to challenge conventional perspectives and promote a most needed dialogue within the profession if we ought to foster social transformation and nurture a community that honors a holistic and ecologically responsible approach to health and well-being.

Nick, Vagner, and Pamela welcomed the challenge of dreaming of a collective book project that can be used in the classroom to ignite the fire within, to think outside of the box, to challenge our colonized minds and bodies to think of our collective good as a fragile species in a planet devastated by our own occupations, with the hopes that, from within, we can weave the fine threads of our fragile existences into a human tapestry open to give and receive warmth, converse, and learn from each other.

The purpose of this book is to allow the stories of Latin American occupational therapists to be told directly by those who live them, lending an authenticity often missing in outsider perspectives. This book captures occupational therapy as practiced within Latin America's living contexts, underscoring experiences rooted in shared struggles, resilience, and a commitment to social justice. This project now includes over 30 authors from 15 Latin American countries, all contributing insights into the culturally grounded practices of occupational therapy across the region.

The book is organized into four thematic parts: "Lifeways," "Identities," "Territories," and "Arenas." Each part symbolizes an element and cardinal point, essential components of human experience worldwide.

In "Lifeways," Chapters 1 and 2 provide a journey through Indigenous perspectives, practices, and principles, establishing occupational therapy as deeply connected to ancestral knowledge and holistic living. Chapter 1 emphasizes the foundational role of Indigenous wisdom in shaping occupational therapy, exploring how groups like the Guaraní, Mapuche, and Kayambi embody cultural resilience and environmental harmony. This chapter highlights the transformative power of understanding traditional ways of life through embedded boxes to reflect and discuss the content connecting with the reader's locality. Chapter 2 delves into *Buen Vivir*, a philosophy drawn from Indigenous communities across Abya Yala, positioning occupational therapy to reconnect with nature and community. By embedding a worldview that values harmony, these chapters encourage readers to honor Indigenous epistemologies and ways of knowing, promoting collective well-being and environmental respect.

"Identities" (Chapters 3–5) examines race, citizenship, and epistemic diversity, illustrating how occupational therapy can contribute to social resistance and transformation. Chapter 3 tackles racism within occupational therapy training, advocating for anti-racist practices that include the cultural knowledge of Black and Indigenous communities. Chapter 4 explores fluid identities through autobiographical narratives as tools for resistance, allowing occupational therapists to reflect on their diverse backgrounds and challenge Eurocentric norms. Chapter 5 examines how local histories and social-political dynamics shape the profession, encouraging readers to appreciate the importance of regional narratives that resist colonial perspectives. These chapters advocate for an inclusive approach that recognizes the necessity of cultural diversity within the field.

In "Territories" (Chapters 6 and 7), the authors address the geographic and sociopolitical factors influencing occupational therapy's evolution in Latin America. Chapter 6 reflects on the expansion of training programs, analyzing how educational initiatives contribute to sustainable professional practices. The chapter highlights the role of outreach and knowledge production, exemplified by the Amaru Network, in fostering a uniquely Latin American approach to occupational therapy. Chapter 7 focuses on migration, examining how occupational therapy can support migrant populations facing discrimination and cultural displacement. Here, practitioners are encouraged to develop intercultural occupation-based interventions that advocate for social integration, human rights, and anti-racism. These chapters exemplify the profession's commitment to contextually relevant and socially just practices.

Finally, "Arenas" (Chapters 8 and 9) critiques neoliberalism's pervasive influence and advocates for expanded global dialogue. Chapter 8 examines how neoliberal policies have turned health services into consumer-driven practices, challenging occupational therapists to resist commodification and support socially responsive, decolonized care. Chapter 9 introduces intercultural translations as a collaborative approach, encouraging exchanges between Global North and South perspectives to address systemic inequalities within the profession. These chapters underscore the need for occupational therapy to move beyond individualistic frameworks, adopting a more globally relevant role that bridges diverse cultural understandings.

Throughout the book there are some case studies, all of which are fictional or about the contributors.

This book offers an essential entry into the rich landscape of Latin American occupational therapy. While not exhaustive, it serves as the first cohesive narrative on Latin American occupational therapy's evolution, challenging prevailing frameworks and inviting future generations of occupational therapists to engage in inclusive, global dialogues essential for the profession's future. By bringing these perspectives into classrooms worldwide, particularly in the Global North, this book seeks to inspire a commitment to social justice, cultural inclusivity, and interregional collaboration in addressing the global challenges we collectively face.

Nicholas Pollard, Pamela Talero Cabrejo, and Vagner Dos Santos

References

Dos Santos, V., & Gallassi, A. (Eds.) (2014). *Questões Contemporâneas da Terapia Ocupacional na América do Sul* (1st edn). CRV.

Dos Santos, V., Muñoz, I., & Farias, M. (Eds.) (2022). *Questões e práticas contemporâneas da terapia ocupacional na América do Sul* (2nd edn). CRV.

Freire, P. (1970). *Pedagogy of the Oppressed.* Seabury Press.

Groh, L. (1966). *Ferdinand Magellan* (A World Explorer Book). Muller.

Waldman, C. (1964). *The Voyages of Christopher Columbus.* Golden Press.

PART 1

LIFEWAYS

CHAPTER 1

Traditional Existences and Their Ways of Life

LEARNING FROM THEIR PRACTICES, PROJECTS, AND POSSIBILITIES FOR OCCUPATIONAL THERAPY

Maria Daniela Corrêa de Macedo, Lincoyan Painemal Morales, and Bryan Esteban Llerena

Abstract

This chapter presents the wealth of knowledge and wisdom of some native social groups systematically oppressed in Latin America and the Global North and South. To do so, we reviewed the history of these Indigenous communities and the interpenetration of knowledge among them through their ways of life. We have reflected on their contributions to occupational therapy and the future of practices and projects based on cultural understanding. This knowledge also provides a conceptual core that emerges from case studies involving occupational therapists whose social identity is aligned with communities historically oppressed by their races/ethnicities. These are critical for the profession's development in Latin America and the Global North and South. This chapter allows readers to understand the negative social and health impact of racism on individuals and groups and how to overcome and produce equitable care and promote social and environmental justice.

Keywords

Indigenous communities; traditional ways; practices; territory; occupational therapy

Learning outcomes

- Acknowledge the diverse knowledge regarding Indigenous communities in Latin America.

- Discuss the different territories and lifestyles to provide a varied and closer understanding of native groups.
- Understand the negative social and health impact of racism on individuals and groups and how to overcome and produce fair care while promoting social and environmental justice.
- Articulate territorial knowledge, practices, and projects reflecting upon their contributions to occupational therapy and the future of practices and projects based on cultural understanding.

Introduction

This chapter arises from a video call meeting among occupational therapists from Brazil, Chile, and Ecuador. The primary objective was exchanging knowledge and insights from interactions with indigenous ethnic groups across these Latin American countries. Despite the diverse worldviews, the shared experiences were deeply rooted in ancestral traditions, offering revelation and authenticity in their essence.

The methodological framework presented in this chapter is conceptualized as a journey through the territorialities, territories, and bodies through the *walk*, *inhabiting*, and *being* of Indigenous peoples. We follow the *walk* and its relations as it pertains to the Guaraní peoples, their territorialities, and occupational therapy; for the *inhabiting* as it relates to the Mapuche peoples, their territorialities, and occupational therapy; and for the *being* as it relates to the body from the Kayambi people's perspective and occupational therapy. These different worldviews provoke reflections into the professional practice of occupational therapy, emphasizing its ties to ancestry, community life, and diversity. They also highlight the importance of an intersectional political position that acknowledges class, race, ethnicity, and gender relations (Ambrosio & Silva, 2022; Gonzalez, 2020). There is a need to shift the perspective toward emphasizing practices rooted in cultural realities with real contextualized possibilities for transformations (Barros, de Almeida, & Vecchia, 2007).

Indigenous peoples descended from the original inhabitants of the Americas who were present in the region long before the arrival of the European incursions in the late 15th century. The American continent, particularly Latin America, is home to a wide diversity of Indigenous peoples and communities. These groups are often referred to as Amerindians, original peoples, or by the name of their ethnicity. This chapter will focus on three distinct groups: the Guaraní (in Brazil), the Mapuche (in Chile), and the Kayambi (in Ecuador).

Figure 1.1 presents a detailed map delineating the locations of Indigenous ethnic groups discussed in the chapter. Each group is distinctly shown based on their respective countries and specific identifications: Kayambi people (Sierra of Ecuador, Quito, Ibarra, Cayambe, and from the East to the West of Napo), Mapuche territory (Central Chile and Argentina), Andinos (Border of Peru, Northern Chile, Bolivia, and Argentina), Tikuna (Border of Colombia, Brazil, and in the Loreto department of Peru), Fueginos (Southern Chile and Argentina), and territories of the Guaraní. This latter group is further subdivided into the Kaiowá (Brazil-Mato Grosso del Sur), the Mbyás, the Nhandéva, the Aché, and the Pay Tavyterás (extending across Brazil, Uruguay, and Paraguay), the Chiriguano (Chaco Region Bolivia), the Guaraní in Paraguay (southern part of the country and its borders), and the Guaraní in Argentina (Buenos Aires, Jujuy, and Salta).

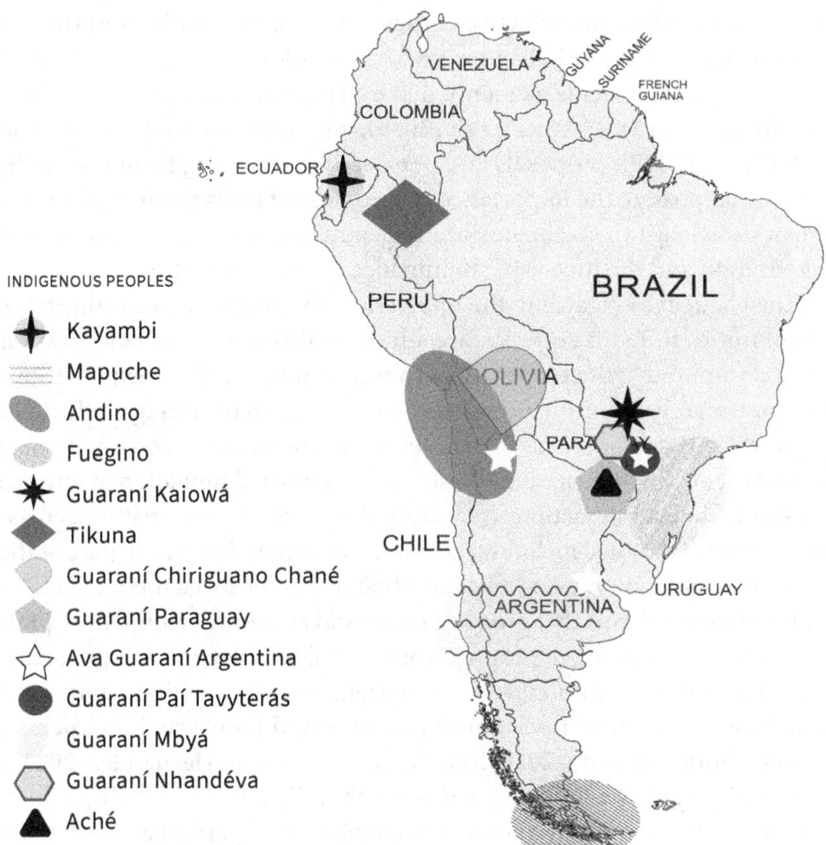

Figure 1.1 Indigenous people's main territories through Latin America (made by Bryan Llerena)

In what follows, we will examine the history of these Indigenous communities and the collective wisdom they have crafted over time. We examine their lifestyle and reflect on their contributions to current and future occupational therapy practices and projects based on cultural and ethnic understanding.

Contextualization of the Indigenous peoples and their struggles in Latin America

Latin America is a geographical framework encompassing different borders, beliefs, cultures, and colonial history. Its histories converge in shared values of solidarity, diversity, and collectivity of Indigenous communities. While it may seem contradictory, such values do not exclude the existence of conflicts but serve to strengthen a sense of community and belonging anchored in collaborative strategies (Macedo, 2016). These strategies have been established in the collective consciousness as mechanisms to survive challenges posed by capitalism, extractivism, colonialism, patriarchy, and even ecological genocide as mentioned by Yrigoyen Fajardo (2009), Simó and Abregú (2015), Milanez et al. (2019), and Krenak (2020). According to Bottinelli (2018), proposals and perspectives emerging from the South not only emphasize the importance of recognizing Indigenous legacies but also acknowledge the resilience of Indigenous communities in the face of colonization and the increasing dominance of Western cultures.

The challenges regarding the oppression and inequality of Indigenous communities in Latin America are a historical result of the colonization process from the 15th century by European countries. These exploitations were not merely about territorial expansion but were strategic efforts to strip Indigenous populations of their territories, principles, goods, and social organization. This violence is not restricted to wars of domination or any one colonizer; violent interactions were created that established a pattern, crossing everyday relations, including economic activities, becoming part of the social structure. Consequently, it seems that spaces for social interaction also evolved into platforms that promote social and ethnic discrimination, prejudice, and racism through programs of internal colonization and genocidal war, often with constitutional change to legitimize these actions, combined with a pattern of colonial relationships that served for extractivist interests of exploitation (Macedo, 2016; Ruiz Guerra & Soriano Hernández, 2023).

Racial prejudice can be defined as a culturally conditioned disposition or attitude that is unfavorable toward members of a particular population based on their physical appearance or the entirety or part of their acknowledged ethnic lineage. Regarding the colonization process in America, Ailton

Krenak, an Indigenous researcher from Brazil, addresses the issue of racism against Indigenous peoples and highlights that:

> this diffuse violence, which remarkably spread across different cosmos, is driven by an inherent inability to accept our differences. The illness of racism, which can be likened to a global epidemic, originated when we separated ourselves from nature to the point where we ceased to share the richness of diversity with nature. Viewing differences as belonging to "The other" created barriers to acceptance. This scenario of seeing diversity as foreign led to the rise of historical racism. Essentially, racism grew from an inability to value differences in others. (Milanez et al., 2019, p. 2172)

The Guaraní, one of Brazil's largest Indigenous populations, mainly inhabits Mato Grosso del Sur and coastal areas. Data from the Brazilian Institute of Geography and Statistics (IBGE, 2010) indicates that over 67,000 identified themselves as Guaraní in the national census, with the Guaraní-Kaiowá subgroup representing more than 43,000. Brand, Colman, and Machado (2008) reported that the Guaraní population in Latin America is approximately 225,000. This includes around 150,000 residing in Bolivia, an estimated 53,500 in Paraguay, and roughly 42,000 in Argentina, with 8000 being Guaraní-Mbya and the rest Ava-Guaraní.

In the 17th century, the Mapuche inhabited the region now identified as southern Chile. They are notable for resisting conquest by the Spanish and the Incas. Historical literature reveals that they began clashing with European invaders from the beginning of 1546, when Pedro de Valdivia entered Chile from the North, crossing the Atacama Desert. He subsequently established the town of Santiago (current capital), expecting a peaceful conquest of the entire region. However, by the 1640s, the Spanish conceded territory to the Mapuche, and only in the 19th century did subsequent Chilean military campaigns invade it again. Despite this, the Mapuche language is not officially recognized in Chile and Argentina, and the resistance movement still exists (Chihuailaf et al., 2012).

The Kayambi people, native to the Ecuadorian Sierra, have gradually lost their territories due to the hacienda system established by the Spaniards and subsequently by the Creoles. This system introduced inhumane treatments through the debt peonage process in everyday life. This contract forced indigenous groups to work in agriculture for a lifetime, hereditarily and with minimal payments (Churuchumbi, 2014). This continued until the 20th century when state institutions furthered deterritorialization to harness natural resources. This exploitation persisted despite indigenous resistance led by figures like Dolores Cacuango and Tránsito Amaguaña (Confederación del Pueblo Kayambi, 2021).

Despite the entire process of genocide and ethnocide of Indigenous communities in Latin America, these groups have shown remarkable resilience. As highlighted by Yrigoyen Fajardo (2009), they have successfully established multifaceted organizational structures in local, national, and regional contexts with a focus on advocacy and ethno-development. In Bolivia, for example, the "Pact of Unity" (2002) was established to facilitate collective action before forums such as the Constituent Assembly, the United Nations system, and international collaborations. This pact brought together four major Indigenous organizations: CIDOB, from the lowlands; Conamaq, from the highlands; the CSUTCB, an organization of colonizing farmers; and Bartolina Sisa, which coordinates women's organizations. Furthermore, international frameworks like the ILO Convention 169 continue to stress the importance of initiatives to fight poverty and unemployment within these Indigenous communities (Yrigoyen Fajardo, 2009).

We propose to review the history of these Indigenous communities and the knowledge fused between them through their ways of life. We reflect on their contributions to professional practice and the future of practices and projects based on cultural and ethnic understanding.

The walk: the *oguata porã* (good walk) and the Guaraní paths

The Guaraní territory in Latin America is presented as a large web shaped by movements, journeys, escapes, quests, needs, desires, and the so-called *oguata porã* (good walk) of these people. These constant motions and walking are central to this group's individual and collective organization that seeks its *ivy marã e'ỹ* (land without evil). This space in this world, which is physical and subjective, allows them to carry out reciprocal relationships, uphold their traditional land occupation, and practice their *nhande reko* (the Guaraní way of life) within these defined territories (Macedo, 2016).

Brand et al. (2008) highlight that the Guaraní language, despite its various dialects, is uniquely spoken across five South American countries. Therefore, Guaraní holds the distinction of being the "historical language" of Mercosur.[1] Observations reveal that irrespective of urban or village settings, the Guaraní organize themselves in networks, building intercultural relationships and cooperative ties. Their emphasis on territorial and geographical connections

1 Mercosur is a South American trade bloc established in 1991 to promote free trade and fluid movement of goods, people, and currency between member countries.

facilitates ongoing interactions, reinforcing their cultural significance and strengthening community unity.

This section explores the Guaraní movements, drawing insights from Macedo's 2016 thesis titled "The Guaraní People of Latin America: Intercultural Relations in Virtual Social Networks and the Construct of Cooperative Networks." These communities' territorial perceptions and organizational methods influence their lifestyles, knowledge, and practices. For those in occupational therapy working alongside Indigenous populations, it is imperative to know these cultural and ethnic distinctions. Such knowledge enriches our professional approach and enhances our relationships with diverse ethnic communities.

The Guaraní movement as a dynamic of personal and collective organization

According to Pissolato (2006), the assertion of Guaraní culture, viewed through the *mbya* perspective of mobility, the *oguata porã* (good walk), is a significant contribution in recent literature. This migrant-religious ethos, intrinsically tied to myth, especially in more contemporary works, tends to be presented in a broader context. It transcends the myth of the land without evil (*yvymarãe'y*) that makes them walk, which would be their "good walk" objective. Instead, it emphasizes an inherent ethos of movement, believed to be instilled by the creators of the Guaraní existence on Earth. This ethos guides their journeys and encapsulates their authentic way of life. It encompasses practices like cultivation and seed dissemination, harmonious coexistence, and the essence of Guaraní spirituality, elements that may appear to be presented collectively or individually.

The Guaraní communities are spread across many municipalities in dozens of villages, further divided into subgroups. Each shows language, ritualistic practices, customs, and political and religious organization differences. An individual from the Guaraní community says on the territory of his people:

> [...]whenever there was a gathering of the Guaraní people there in Paraguay, it always said that there is [...] that trade network between Paraguay, Brazil [...] Mercosur. So, we try to have a network because there was never a border for us. So we wanted to be in contact with the Guaraní people here and there in Paraguay, Argentina, and Bolivia [...] we will continue fighting and discussing [...] because these borders were created by the juruá,[2] it was not by God, like "Ah, from here to there is Paraguay, from here to there is

2 Non-Indigenous.

> Argentina, from here to there is Brazil," it was not God who said that. (Wera Kwaray/Guaraní Mbyá Brazil cited in Macedo, 2016, p. 62)

Teao (2015) recognizes the profound importance of territory to the Guaraní; he analyzes the construction of the Guaraní territory as both physical and imaginary. They are drawn to specific spaces for survival, particularly villages within the Atlantic Mata[3] and near the sea. These locations are often chosen based on religious and mythical elements, manifested through dreams and divine revelations to their leaders. The "imagined territory" concept emerges as these people share an ethnic bond with other Guaraní across the nation, especially in spaces they inhabit, such as villages, museums, schools, and universities. Within these spaces, the Guaraní continuously reshape their collective identities and narratives. The movement between their native villages and these spaces fosters interactions, evident in visits, rituals, seed exchanges, marriages, and political alliances. Such movements strengthen their shared cultural feelings and help them redefine their physical and imaginary sense of territory.

Regarding the dynamics of the Guaraní lifestyle, Pissolato (2006) argues that pathways and walking are central to the Guaraní identity, shaping their mobility, sociability, and individual identity. Concerning mobility observed among the Mbyá communities, the author comments that such phenomena are deeply intertwined with religious beliefs. This is directly associated with the myth of the quest for *yvymarãe'y* (land without evils), a religiosity driven by the promise of what can be achieved beyond this life. This belief forms their migratory patterns, especially toward the Atlantic, perceived as closer to this sacred land. Silva (2007) introduces a transformative perspective, illustrating Guaraní's spatial mobility as a tangible manifestation of human experience, essential for preserving their cultural essence. However, the disputes of private land ownership and subsequent disputes in the postcolonial era of America have rendered such mobility practices increasingly difficult and challenging[4] for the Guaraní to sustain (Glauser & Villagra, 2020).

Across regions in Brazil, Argentina, and Paraguay, the Guaraní have displayed a distinct networked dynamic, as observed in the fieldwork of this study. This dynamic is characterized by seed exchanges, marriages, and migrations,

3 The Atlantic Forest located between Brazil, Paraguay, and Argentina.

4 Glauser and Villagra (2020) discuss contemporary processes of dispossession and re-territorialization affecting the Ava Guaraní, Mbya Guaraní, and Pae Tavyterã peoples in the Eastern Region of Paraguay. In the context of discussing mobility practices and land ownership disputes, the Guaraní peoples in Paraguay are facing significant challenges in maintaining their traditional territories and ways of life. These challenges are likely due to various factors, such as encroachment by non-Indigenous settlers, economic development projects, or changes in land use policies.

reflecting sociability deeply rooted in their original group and reinterpreted within the context of newer groups. While several motivations can instigate these mobility patterns, kinship is consistently emphasized to guide these movements. Even for short-term territorial settlements, the Guaraní often rely on the communities and homes of their relatives (Macedo, 2016).

> Therefore, "mobility" is a new word. Prior to the arrival of the whites, there were no municipalities, states, or countries, and in all these places, Guaraní peoples walked freely (without anyone saying anything) because they were in their territory, in their own world. In the same way, today, a person (Guaraní) can be in Florianópolis, and after a few days in São Paulo or Paraná, we say this person is in the same place, in a single territory. But the whites do not understand this. (Ladeira & Tupã, 2004, p. 59)

There is a noticeable decline in the demarcation of Indigenous territories (capitalist interests are seeking to absorb and exploit the natural environment both through legal and illicit means) as the Indigenous population witnesses significant growth, leading to territorial disputes and challenges in maintaining their traditional lifestyles. The years 2013 and 2014 were characterized by significant protests and campaigns, predominantly on social media platforms, favoring the cause of Indigenous land demarcation. While support for the Indigenous cause emerged across various sectors of civil society, negotiations with landowners and the state's inclination toward agribusiness seem endless. In addition, the ongoing efforts of the National Congress to amend the existing legislation on land demarcation in Brazil further complicate territorial management.

This community persistently seeks ways to reorganize and adapt the Guaraní way of life. Within these dynamics, occupational therapists and the Indigenous community can learn and derive meaning from their intercultural and interethnic engagements and mediations (Macedo et al., 2016).

The Researcher's Path and the Guataha Condition: A Case Study

The field visits to the Guaraní communities undertaken during the research leading to Macedo's 2016 thesis are reported here. It illustrates reflections on the Guaraní way of life and their relationship with their territory.

Walking through various Guaraní territories and symbolizing the *guataha*, representing a "wanderer" as Silva (2007) described, the researcher perceived variances in their societal structures, influenced by spatial, temporal, and locational factors. A remarkable experience was addressing Guaraní adaptability in urban contexts, strategic shifts, and identity resignifications. These communities, irrespective of their geographical placements, radiated a harmonious synchronicity. The research journey for the collection of research data began in Argentina, marked by participation in the *ara pyahu* (new year) ritual, the *mbaraka* or Guaraní maraca (rattle) was played, and they blew and smoked all together with their *petynguá* (pipe). Traditional Guaraní rituals, instruments, and symbols were prominently featured, such as the *takuapu*, a musical instrument only played by women, the *mbaraka*, and others, such as flowers, Andean fabrics, burning herbs like an incense burner, and the Wiphala flag (symbol of the Andean peoples).

The researcher relates how he met a Guaraní elder who told his story and the life of Avá Guaraní: We sat down and introduced ourselves better. "I talked about my work with the Guaraní in Brazil. He spoke of his community *Ywy Memby* (children of the earth), in La Plata, on the outskirts of the state of Buenos Aires, a little far from the capital, and then asked me if I was Catholic because he wanted to emphasize 'the atrocities that Christians had already committed throughout world history.' I replied that I was from a Catholic family." He continued to recount that he was taken from his community by the Jesuits and had a very hard childhood, as they forbade him to speak and sing in Guaraní, but he said that all he knew was how to sing. He suffered many reprimands and punishments for humming in his language. With a look of great pain and suffering, he said that they had taken everything from him because, over time, he no longer knew how to speak his language and much less hum his sacred songs. "I was moved by Gumercindo's story." He continued talking about his pain from not living with his people and having been forced to learn other things and how much this left him with a huge void, no longer knowing who he was in his childhood. He learned trades, moved to the city, started a family, and finally managed to build that community. However, he pointed out that they suffer from neglect and poverty, as well as living with the prejudice of being Indigenous but not a real Guaraní because he had been forced to abandon Guaraní ways and culture. "With each sentence, he filled me with emotion; his words were full of wisdom, and he pronounced them with a clear tone of voice and in perfect Spanish." We did not get to know his community. Still, the feelings of pain and strength, transmitted through his words and gestures, "made me understand how cruel the Jesuit missions and the colonization process of America seemed to me, a story that was no longer in books and articles, but it was there, so real and emotive. A quick but very intense gathering that filled me and disturbed me for several moments of my stay in Argentina and Paraguay, a blend of compassion, revolt, pain, disbelief, belief, faith, strength, but with whom? Everything was adding up facts, stories, and emotions, and my beliefs were being affected, my way of being, my path."

These groups constantly experience both genocide and ethnocide. They suffer a cultural erasure of their identity and lifestyle, and they are at constant risk of survival. In Jasy Porã, a village located in northeastern Argentina, the community leader guided us through the village and began to talk about Guaraní knowledge. He spoke of the need to revalue nature again as the only path to survive on Earth. If there are rivers, forests, and birds, there is strength, too; the energy of nature is side by side with the gods and in everyone's heart, giving us the will to live and ensuring the Earth is a better place to live. But today, it is a bit difficult; without nature, no Guaraní would survive, because when nature is lost, strength is also lost. This path was marked by numerous gatherings and exchanges, leading to a deeper understanding of the dynamic processes that shape the Guaraní individuals, the community, and the broader ethnic group. These processes manifest in their movements, wanderings, and ability to find and connect with others. Even in the most challenging circumstances, they intensify and practice relationships based on solidarity and unity. The Guaraní's social interactions transform, and through these reinterpretations, new networks of social and territorial relationships are reconstructed across Latin American territories.

Reflective questions

- How might the Guaraní worldview and their lifestyles shape occupational therapy practices?
- Why are the knowledge and practices of a community vital for the professional practice of occupational therapy?
- How does territory impact the human occupations of the individuals in this region?
- How does the Guaraní act of walking shape the life projects of these wanderers? And how has this also influenced the researcher's experience?

The path is shaped by walking

In the Guaraní perspective and worldview, territory is not dissociated from the physical, human, subjective, and spiritual elements. Instead, these represent a lineage, ensuring the continuity of the ethnic group. Movement, migration, and walking are vital in establishing a reciprocity, solidarity, and communal identity network. Important elements of the culture determine the activities, knowledge, and roles the community will maintain or reinterpret, considering the path that can be forged individually or collectively.

Regarding professional practice, particularly when it pertains to territorial relevance and significance to a specific group or individual, it is imperative for occupational therapists to develop culturally relevant activities for the community. This involves how the most valued activities within the community are perceived and how they align with the key symbols shaping identities. Therefore, it is essential that occupational therapists create interventions that are congruent with specific local cultures, departing from actions governed by conventional technical procedures. This approach stresses the concept of "otherness," a relational notion cultivated through dialogue (Barros et al., 2007).

Within cultural practice, a primary challenge is facilitating spaces that foster interaction and discourse among diverse ethnic communities. Cultural mediation emphasizes collaborative efforts aimed at addressing and responding to various demands, from resistance and conflict resolution to even the reinforcement of ethnic identities in the face of ethnocide. Drawing from the Guaraní perspective, it is pertinent to highlight that challenges are often solved, underscoring the idea that the path is indeed forged as one walks along.

Inhabiting: Exploring Mapuche territory and territoriality

As a result of the interactions between the Mapuche and the Western Chilean societies, a clear disparity in their respective conceptualizations of "territory" becomes apparent. On the one hand, for the Mapuche community, the term "territory" encompasses not just the geographical dimension but also the sociocultural and the spiritual-immaterial realms wherein life manifests (Bengoa, 1996).

From the indigenous perspective, the concept of territory is intrinsically linked to the genesis of the cosmos, including its vertical and horizontal dimensions, as will be explained. Central to this understanding is the element of spirituality. Therefore, the cosmogonic and cosmological frameworks that define the territory illustrate its organization. This organization reveals specific structures, forms, and norms that serve as foundational principles governing Indigenous peoples and their interactions with their surroundings. These guiding principles bestow meaning upon the notions of place, spatiality, land, and territory (Zapata, 2010).

Within the Western paradigm, territory is, by contrast, perceived as the tangible space inhabited by specific human groups. This space is viewed as a tangible asset, subject to claims of ownership. It is seen as a domain that can be cultivated, and its natural assets can be exploited for economic production. Furthermore, this perspective emphasizes the establishment of individual, corporate, and governmental dominion over the territory (Renard, 2009; Rodríguez Valbuena, 2010).

Thereupon, differences arise between Mapuche and Western understandings concerning territory, leading to an epistemological disagreement in ways of knowing, understanding, interacting, and utilizing its natural resources (Tubino, 2014).

This section represents an initial exploration into the concepts of territory and territoriality, as perceived through the Mapuche worldview. It serves as a starting point to address topics related to habitation and occupation, which unveils new spaces for occupational therapy.

First approach: The Mapuche perspective

In the culture of the Mapuche people, the term *mapu* is polysemous, commonly translated as "land" in the Western context. Those who reside on this land are termed *mapu-che* (people of the land), and their spoken language, *mapu-(n)-dungu(n)*, translates to "the language of the land." However, from the Mapuche worldview, territory transcends mere geographical boundaries. It incorporates the spaces historically inhabited by communities in an objective and subjective relationship. This individualistic and collective bond holds the relationship of spirituality and reciprocity as essential (Quintriqueo et al., 2018–2021).

Territory is conceptualized as a multidimensional space constructed over time. This territorial notion carries profound epistemological implications, transcending mere physical confines, and is conceived in vertical and horizontal relationships.

The vertical dimension (*wenu mapu*) refers to a higher space upheld by spiritual forces; the horizontal dimension (*nag mapu*) refers to the earth and its territory, where physical and biological life is generated; and the notion of inferior dimension (*minche mapu*) refers to the forces that support life beneath the earth's surface (Millán et al., 2021). This analysis primarily focuses on the *nag mapu* dimension, where each person (*che*) lives, even though this dimension is indivisible from the others.

In this degree, human-inhabited spaces emerge from intricate relationships woven daily between individuals, nature, societal structures, and the cosmogonic conception of time. Essentially, to grasp the notion of territory (*mapu*), the concepts of the land–man–nature relationship must be understood, that is, how the *che* (human) is positioned on the *mapu* (land). This process is different and unique across various spaces or territories, raising their own distinct characteristics. Likewise, understanding the notion of *che* (person) remains elusive without contextualizing it within the *mapu* (territory). This is because it is a human condition situated in a particular space, laden with an ethical, value-based, normative, and knowledge-driven framework that one must achieve throughout life concerning a defined territory (*lof, rewe*).

Consequently, distinct regions within the *mapu* are designated based on geographical positioning. The inhabitants, in turn, derive their nomenclature from these locales. For instance, *lafken* signifies marine territory characterized primarily by its natural attributes. Its denizens are termed *lafken-che*, translating to the people of the *lafken* (sea or lake). Thus, a series of relationships is constructed between people and their territories, culminating in diverse territorial identities such as *huilli-che* (inhabitant of the south) and *pewen-che* (mountain range inhabitants).

In summary, the territorial concept denotes relational aspects, suggesting ties of dominion, power, belonging, or ownership between specific geographical spaces and individual or collective entities. Under this premise arises the notion of *wall-mapu* (all the land, integrally), which connects these social relationships' material and symbolic dimensions.

Territoriality, as a concept, alludes to specific behaviors exhibited within a territory that relate to how one comes to inhabit and remain in space. This space is governed by distinct life rhythms and interactions with the environment and other inhabitants, which may vary in similarities and differences. In essence, through their interactions with the environment and its inherent diversities, humans claim spaces, determine routes, mark territories, and imprint their distinct signatures upon nature.

Likewise, such territories function as symbolic spaces. Their significance is not confined merely to their material attributes. They transcend the mere act of occupying a physical space, transforming every human dimension into potential habitats. This transformation is contingent upon someone who expresses, conceptualizes, or envisions the characteristics of the space. For Indigenous communities, the subjective and intersubjective facets of space and time are central to constructing a comprehensive worldview. Such insights offer a unique way of seeing and understanding reality, serving as a specific epistemic result. This perspective is a foundational framework for the Mapuche lifeworld's existential and experiential background (Quintriqueo et al., 2018–2021).

Second approach: Inhabiting the territory

The word "inhabit" is defined as the act of residing or dwelling within a place or space. Humans inhabit places, establishing relationships and experiences within those places and shaping their daily lives. In other words, inhabitation means the relationship forged between individuals and their living space (Giglia, 2012).

In the Mapuche worldview, inhabitation emerges from the relationship between territory and life. Discussing the concept of territory (*mapu*) means talking about life (*mongen*) in its various manifestations and visible and non-visible present expressions. Therefore, *mongen* is present in every facet of *mapu*, and without *mapu*, there is no *mongen*. The *mapu*, in essence, compresses and sustains all existential entities. However, in its interaction with the *che* (person), there must be a specific order, a set of ethical guidelines, values, and a regulated way of interacting. These rules come from the Mapuche's understanding of their origins and are summarized in their *azmapu* or Mapuche Law (Melín, Mansilla, & Royo, 2017).

For life (*mongen*) to thrive, there is a crucial emphasis on balance between humanity and nature, interacting within the fundamental principle of *kelluwun* (reciprocity). The Mapuche way of life is based on the principle that everything is interconnected somehow; nothing exists in isolation. This philosophy states that each person establishes their own way of inhabiting, as no two places or people are identical, and thus, no two ways of inhabiting those places can be the same. There is no pre-established way to inhabit; each human being chooses and creates their own way of doing it.

The act of inhabitation is related to being, staying, or living in a place. It connects to time, duration, moments of pause, or lingering. To inhabit transcends the simplistic notion of mere occupancy; it expresses the deeper connection of appropriating a place where individuals express themselves, a process in which the inhabited space becomes a repository for the traces or marks of life.

To inhabit the world is acknowledging a specific territory as a constitutive part of our identity. It is about giving meaning to the objects around us. Nevertheless, this notion transcends mere physicality, related to the feelings of rootedness, belonging, and emotional attachment that individuals feel toward their inhabited spaces. This feeling is inevitably linked to the physical and sociocultural world they are part of. Through this perspective, individuals find fulfillment by belonging to and growing within a place.

Third approach: To inhabit is to occupy

As mentioned, inhabiting is the relationship between an individual and their living space; it expresses our way of being (or living) on Earth. In this context, inhabiting is both a doing (an activity) and a way of being, which bridges the practical and existential dimensions. In this way, rethinking this relationship between humans and their environment leads to an understanding that inhabiting is not limited to the local and restricted boundaries of living in the world but highlights the connection to the world itself.

Inhabiting a territory means walking, engaging with, sharing, and understanding it. Inhabiting the world implies a dependency on others. In this sense, to inhabit is to participate and connect uniquely. It involves the recovery of one's own inner freedom. It means learning to listen and share, free from predefined fear, conclusion, belief, or judgment. Inhabiting is walking, moving, and displacing, lingering upon a space. It is idling time, warming up under the sun. It is about contemplation, resting, and breathing. It is free time.

Inhabiting allows people to construct a memory and a projection. Memory is related to personal and interpersonal history, the trajectory and belonging to a family or community. Through these memories, people connect with and give meaning to their surroundings.

About the Mapuche worldview
Reflective questions

- How should we understand the notion of territory and forms of appropriation?
- How is territoriality expressed in terms of human habitation?
- How is human habitation visualized in terms of occupation?
- How do we exercise disciplinary praxis in a culturally relevant way?

A final approach: A necessary provocation

Within the Latin American context, occupational therapy has been evolving its disciplinary praxis from a territorial and intersectoral perspective aligned with social issues. This evolution has resulted in the term "community area," recognizing that individuals interact with others and that the person is anchored to the world of life and the system world in a dialogical, irreversible, historical, situated way.

Drawing from this theoretical positioning, various perspectives emerge concerning the concept of territory. In Chile, Pino Morán, Ceballos Concha, and Sepúlveda Hernández (2015) assert that people are ontologically communal and occupational. They argue that individuals are anchored in the world of life, which encompasses the everyday experience, common sense, and the communal world, a primary concern for this dimension of occupational therapy.

On the other hand, within the Colombian context and aligning with this conceptual trajectory, Garcia (2014) suggests the territory as an entity shaped (and reshaped) by historical narratives, aspirations, prevailing power dynamics, and lives intertwined therein. Similarly, Rojas Castillo et al. (2019) elucidate a perspective of territory as an ever-evolving sociocultural construct ceaselessly transformed by communities. These communities, in turn, find themselves in an ongoing fight against authoritative structures, such as the government.

Paraphrasing the meaning of the premise proposed by Pino et al. (2015), we suggest that human existence is ontologically territorial and occupational since it is within the territory, place, or inhabited space where people construct, reconstruct, or deconstruct their life experiences.

Thus, the notion that territory and occupation are relational phenomena is deeply embedded in cultural facts. Humans inhabit and appropriate a space/time, manifesting both material and symbolic doings. So, inhabiting inherently implies occupation, an understanding inextricably linked to the habits, routines, and competencies spread over time.

Territoriality, conceptualized as ways of living and habitation, means establishing various connections, such as events. From this perspective, territory emerges as a collective construct, a dialogue between human beings and nature throughout history. Over millennia, early human societies have concentrated their collective efforts toward forging a cohesive society, an economy, a culture, and an identity associated with a specific place. This "place" is understood as a space of appropriation, which serves as a reference point for understanding the territory, facilitating symbolic and identitarian reference.

There is a close relationship between inhabiting and living. To inhabit this world means giving significance to the objects surrounding us. Inhabitation means recognizing a territory as an integral part of our identity. Humans emerge as architects of the countless scenarios that make up their environment. They are seen as builders breathing life and purpose into spaces and objects.

From an occupational therapy perspective, addressing the process of inhabitation in terms of territoriality necessitates a multifaceted exploration. This exploration addresses the dynamics of relationships individuals foster with spaces, explained in three important dimensions: the intrapersonal, the interpersonal, and the environmental. Each person belongs to a specific time and place; they navigate their own life, becoming aware of the place they inhabit; they designate and recognize the territory where they carry out their daily tasks, giving it a feeling of rootedness, belonging, and attachment. In essence, human beings are intrinsically territorial entities who transform the Earth to make it their home, and in this transformative act, humans also undergo changes. These changes are also shaped by the land's effects on human beings and their society.

Accordingly, we can reflect on how cultural groups have become inhabitants and the impacts made on their daily lives and ways of living and being.

Being: Corporeality within the Kayambi people's perspective

The way of living in the Kayambi community also has different principles from those found in Western knowledge, aligning with the Andean worldview. This perspective captures how the relationship between humans, nature, and the cosmos is perceived and felt (Chimbolema, 2017). This intricate relationship is further delineated through various elements and principles, as presented in Table 1.1.

Table 1.1 Elements of Andean cosmology (Achig-Balarezo, 2019)

Element	Concept
Equality	Within the interpretation of the world, each element is not self-sufficient but exists in a symbiotic relationship, each needing mutual reliance for survival.
Time-cyclicity	Time is not perceived linearly segmented into past, present, and future. Instead, it is categorized as a cyclical spiral, where the past is seen as a point from which one moves forward and backward. This is represented in the spiral that interconnects the different times.
Holism	The principle is that everything that makes up *pachamama*, whether a living being or inherent, is as important as any other. Each being is part of a greater whole.
Immanence	Within the Andean world, everything is perceived, even if it is not material, such as rivers, mountains, the air, the earth, etc.
Reciprocity	Expressed at a pragmatic and ethical level where every action is seen as a cosmic contribution, it embodies the principle of giving to receive.
Complementarity	Including complementary opposites that form an integral whole, such as woman–man, night–light, and sun–moon.
Pachamama	*Pacha* means time-space, and *mama* is mother. *Pachamama* is a living being. It involves all levels of the cosmos and moves through dimensions of the upper plane, this world, the intermediary, and the underworld, which are cosmic and telluric forces from different worlds, all of which are in the Andean worldview.

Everyday life in the Kayambi community

Within the Kayambi community, thinking and working are the same, and there is no division between the mind and body (Farinango, 2020). The daily tasks are built collectively as a strategy against violating rights. This is manifested through cooperative economic systems, community assemblies, Indigenous justice, and reciprocity. As articulated by Mama Tránsito Amaguaña, "unity is like the cob; if the grain goes away, the row goes away; if the row goes away, the cob ends" (Confederación del Pueblo Kayambi, 2021).

In the Kayambi people, there is a pronounced emphasis on collective occupations, which can be traced back to ancestral traditions. These practices serve as an insurgent value against neoliberal capitalism, often marked by individualism, immediacy, hedonism, and competitiveness (Churuchumbi, 2014). Among the Kayambi, there are some common collective practices, such as the *minka*, agroecological *chakras*, and community assemblies. *Minka* is an organization of people with a common goal (Cruz, 2018). The *chakra* is a common space to share and interact with nature, where the diversity, solidarity, and abundance of *pachamama* are palpable.

Engaging with and reflecting upon community perspectives offers a transformative and enriching experience. This is exemplified in the case of Blanca, a mother and grandmother, and her daughter and grandson, who have intellectual disabilities. She imparts wisdom from her multifaceted *chakra*, illustrating a harmonious ecosystem. Blanca relates the diversity of *pachamama* through the intrinsic behaviors and identities of individuals. Through her insights, it is possible to understand how the *chakra* integrates her family members with disabilities into the community.

The *chakana*: A convergence of health, illness, and ancestral knowledge of the body

The human body, a repository of life's events, is subject to diverse interpretations regarding its existence. Within the Kayambi community, the body transcends mere annexation to nature, collective consciousness, and the soul. Instead, it is perceived as a territory where full existence is expressed. Hence, health, body, and existence intertwine with food, space, community, and nature, which converge in the *chakana* (Rengifo, 2018).

The *chakana*, derived from the term *tawa chakana*, translates to "four stairs," while *pusi chakani* signifies "four bridges." This symbology holds maximum significance in Andean culture, composed of a series of concepts from the indigenous communities of the Central Andes. This region witnessed the flourishing of the Inca Empire and its antecedent pre-Inca cultures, including the Kayambi community. The *chakana* is related to the Andean culture's spirituality, philosophy, and science, containing the interconnections between worlds, values, geo-biodiversity, flora, fauna, sacred times, sensory perception, feelings, flavors, organs, and guiding values. This is further harmonized with the natural elements (earth, water, fire, air, and wood) (Rengifo, 2018). The *chakana* expresses the harmonious balance that moves in the body, intertwining dietary habits, emotional states, and the relationship with nature and its community (see Figure1.2). Within this paradigm, "health" is perceived as the harmonious nexus between nature, oneself, and the broader community (Confederación del Pueblo Kayambi, 2021).

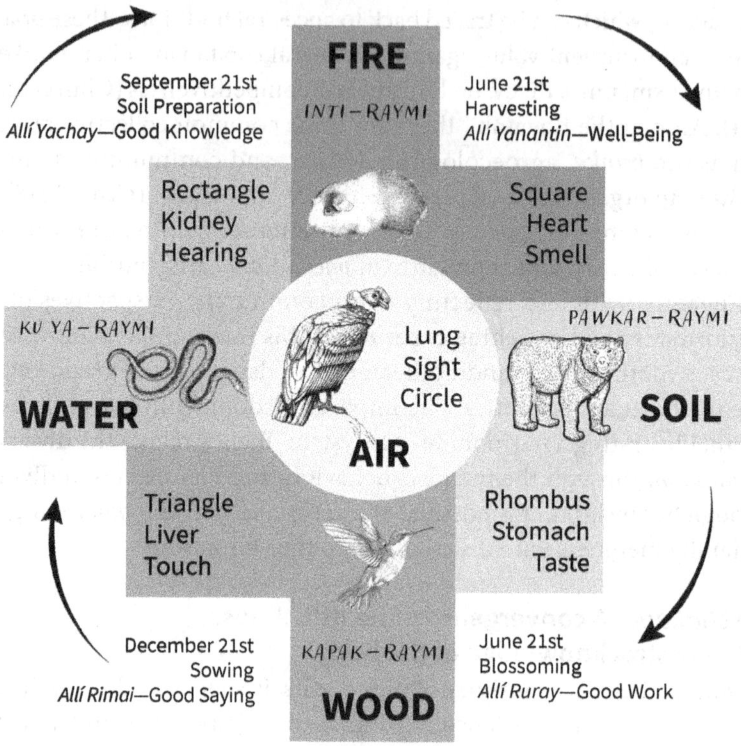

Figure 1.2 The *chakana* as represented by the Kayambi community (made by Bryan Llerena)

Note: The dates of sacred *raymi* celebrations are related to the elements and actions for the prosperity of agricultural products alongside the foundational principles and values gathered in the *alli* worldview. This connection extends further to the organs and senses, presenting a ladder of concepts that underpins the balance of health in nature, the community, and the individual body.

The conceptualization of illness aligns with the foundational principles of occupational therapy, emphasizing the connection between the mind and body and acknowledging the subjectivity of the mind (Gálvez, Godoy, & Lagos, 2010). The disease is perceived as a malevolent entity or a state of parity (Fabio, 2010), manifesting as a socio-cosmic disequilibrium. This imbalance engenders conflict, altercations, and health disturbances, often stemming from violating millennial precepts related to justice and social collectivity. Within this duality of health and illness, the essence of life is experienced through the paradigms of *sumak kawsay* and *alli kawsay* (Laverde, 2001).

Sumak kawsay means a life characterized by fulfillment and harmony, while *alli kawsay* expresses good daily living. Central to these concepts is the pursuit of prosperity between humans and nature, valuing creativity, collective work, cooperation, and exchange. The importance of "sharing" is emphasized, and citizen participation organization is highlighted (Churuchumbi, 2014).

Taking the position of decolonial occupational therapy helps us perceive and understand the experiences of *sumak kawsay* and *alli kawsay* as professionals. This paradigm challenges traditional thinking based on moral, political, and cultural beliefs. It adopts an ethical-political-cultural position, providing eyes, language, and hands to communicate and share the existence of a body intricately interconnected with nature and the collective.

The principles of the Andean worldview need to be understood in people's daily lives as they create bridges to form a path and support the development of strategies from an ethnic-occupation perspective, a relativistic position of occupation linked to ethical and political commitment. Zango Martín and Moruna Mirales (2013) conducted an analysis on the observation of games among infants in Bolívar, Ecuador. The study identified challenges in the approach to the number of users in childcare centers and the little importance that relatives give to games. This leaves children in a liminal space devoid of recreational opportunities. There is a pressing need for practices that provide a dialogue of knowledge, generate peer-to-peer interactions, and emphasize cycles and specific spaces. Such practices should encourage critical and reflective thinking, positioning occupational therapy as a tool of liberation from everyday life oppression, and promoting democracy and the common good (Simó, 2018); this can be exemplified by granting voice to the children in the Bolívar-Ecuador community. This can be further understood by examining how the Andean worldview influences Juan's life in the following case study.

The Kayambi Case

The community of Quito Loma is located on the upper slopes of the inter-Andean basins, surrounded by great mountains, crossed by stoned roads. The houses are made of concrete blocks and have a single room; each home has its agricultural plot. The community has electricity and water from the multiple reservoirs and channels they have built. Notably, there are a few light poles and no telephone signal. Public transportation is limited, with a distinct green bus making its rounds three to four times daily. The primary agricultural activities are cultivating long onions, potatoes, and melloco (a kind of tuber) and raising poultry, cows, and sheep. Quito Loma is built collaboratively by all the families of the community. A school marks the community's downtown, the community gathering house, and a soccer field grazed by different animals from the community.

Juan is a 59-year-old farmer who is happy to raise and care for his laying hens and agricultural plots of white onions. He is proud of his agroecological *chakra* (a diversified food cultivation). Juan and his family actively participate in community activities. Juan has hearing and intellectual disabilities. He lives in a house with his brothers, cousins, mother, uncles, and nephews. For personal hygiene, he uses pots of hot water. His home consists of a single room with noticeable dirt on his bed, floor, and clothes. Regarding community engagements, he contributes to local logistics, such as road construction, participates in celebrations, and offers harvests to divine entities. Once, specialists from the USA evaluated Juan. Their assessments identified problems related to his unfamiliarity with sign language, illiteracy, personal hygiene, community interactions, clothing hygiene difficulties, and home management issues, particularly observing dirt on his clothes, bed, and home, in addition to his disability. However, this assessment might overlook the cultural significance of the soil, crops, and their role in Juan's life.

Reflection questions

- From the Andean worldview, which emphasizes harmonious coexistence with one's surroundings, community, and self, which tenets and facets of the Andean cosmology resonate in Juan's narrative and the ethos of his community?
- Given Juan's profound connection with the land, and considering *pachamama* and the principle of immanence, what might be the underlying reasons for Juan's intentional incorporation of soil in his home, bed, and clothes? If the soil is esteemed as a sentient entity that nurtures and surrounds us, could its presence in everyday spaces, such as sleeping or within one's abode, bear profound significance?

Drawing from Juan's case and the contexts of the children in Bolívar, it becomes evident that occupational therapists must approach the realities of the individuals we engage with. It is imperative to create connections that facilitate understanding a community intricately connected with its environment. By equipping ourselves with discerning perspectives, communication, and skills, we can truly understand the diversity of existence. This approach supports the visibility of a body in harmony with nature and community as a tool for transformation and an inclusive proposal for individuals living in diverse circumstances.

Revealing the walk, the inhabiting, and the being: Potential pathways for learning and engagement in occupational therapy

Considering the construction and realization of actions by the occupational therapist in various cultural contexts, particularly in societies marked by inequalities and oppressions, it is necessary to understand the history and the national sociopolitical-economic and cultural scenario, especially within the plan of social rights. The occupational therapist's work in the context of culture with Indigenous peoples in Brazil has been built through practices and reflections, constantly surrounded by dilemmas and challenges. These practices involve working with different ethnicities in various contexts, combining them in multiple creative actions when encountering the "other," using resources collectively constructed within the communities.

Drawing from the experiences of Guaraní women, we highlight their engagements in self-care activities, particularly emphasizing their use of herbs and medicinal plants. Intriguingly, many traditional caregiving methods have evolved, leading to a profound realization of the diminished use of certain herbs. Beyond their cleansing properties akin to soap, these herbs also offered spiritual protection (Macedo et al., 2021).

In this context, while it is feasible to undertake cultural interventions across diverse groups via occupational therapy within cultural contexts, in the intricate dynamics of the social organization of ethnic groups, ethnic action is also proposed—specific actions related to ethnic groups and the dynamics of ethnicity. Problems can arise related to the social organization and ethnic belonging of groups due to the power dynamics between cultures, such as domination, prejudice, racism, hierarchical delineation of experiences and learnings, spatiality, territoriality, territorial organization, ecological considerations, and even extending to negotiations within ethnic boundaries (Macedo et al., 2016).

In outreach and research projects, experiences and narratives highlight the distinct demands and necessities inherent to the sociocultural organization and differentiation of the Guaraní communities in Latin America.

For the Mapuche community, the conceptualization of territorial habitation transcends mere physicality. It deals with a holistic perspective between humans, nature, and how the cosmos is perceived and understood. This worldview posits the universe and different worlds on different planes that interconnect existing varied planes, each connected within unique philosophical ideologies and worldviews. This perspective involves the constructs individuals formulate regarding the spatial conditions represented in the territory. In essence, it contains several emotions, feelings, symbols, experiences, desires, and dreams. Such a confluence ensures that the inhabited space becomes an intrinsic part of one's being and, to a certain extent, an integral facet of one's personal and societal identity.

For the Kayambi community, embracing the insights derived from their unique worldview and understanding the corporeal existence not only augments but also humanizes and enriches the occupational therapy practice. It positions occupational therapy as a transformative instrument, advocating for the inclusion of bodies within these parties. This worldview perspective prompts reflection, urging us to contemplate the profound interconnectedness of the territory, mountains, food, animals, and the community and how these elements are assimilated and internalized within the human form, fostering critical thoughts and dialogues. Regarding interculturality, remaining receptive to proposals and approaches rooted in collective knowledge becomes crucial, thereby solidifying a decolonial political view.

Inside the worldview perspective of Indigenous communities, the conceptualization surrounding "territory" is linked with constructs associated with space; terms such as places, sites, and landscapes, among others, are connected to a spatial condition that seems essential in people's lives.

In summary, the territory is a multidimensional construct whose meaning is built and consolidated permanently from social, economic, and political processes. Therefore, any discourse on territory involves reviewing various aspects and thinking and organizing several elements to approach a constantly evolving concept. Fundamentally, the territory is a construct intrinsically linked to the individual, applying a profound influence on all associated processes and endeavors.

Territoriality, alternatively termed territorialization, comprises the act of ascribing significance to a territory, facilitated through the habits, practices, and customs of an individual or a collective subject. Territorialization is associated with a process in which a subject, community, or social group appropriates and connects with a physical place. Different experiences, memories, and the semiotic production of the inhabitants at a specific moment characterize this bond.

Dynamics of dominion and power emerge through the interactions of individuals with other people whose sociocultural matrices are different and even divergent within a territory. This dynamic results from the asymmetrical relationships resulting from historical processes of invasion and colonialism on this continent. In this context, territories emerge as expressions of power relations that establish norms, define boundaries, and determine who belongs or is excluded from a particular place. However, it is vital to acknowledge that political processes neither begin nor end with states. In this encounter/mismatch around habitation, practices of resistance, adaptation, and negotiation arise that persist over time.

Nevertheless, an interesting perspective pertinent to occupational therapy relates to living and inhabiting a territory. From this perspective, everyday practices are positioned at the centre of the territorial experience, aiming to identify those behaviors, actions, and gestures. These can range from the subtle to the overt and might frequently manifest in repetitive patterns. Through these actions, people interact with their surroundings in various ways, from making spaces their own to assigning functions, avoiding, or even transforming them physically and symbolically.

In this area, an important element in understanding the territory is the emotions and the emotional link established with it. These emotions are linked to the construction of both personal and social identity, the establishment of relationships, the construction of community, and experiences and living, which become part of what each subject represents in the space they inhabit. To approach the reading of the relationships of affection and the affective links that are established with the territory, it is essential to approach the notion of the concept of community from the perspective of the native peoples, whose viewpoint is profoundly biocentric, and from this, to try to establish a basis for analyzing the relationships between the inhabitants of a territory, which are undoubtedly complex and particular.

From the occupational therapy perspective, the territory cannot be conceived as something natural, as it manifests itself as a social product given from the constructions that go beyond the physical space inhabited by someone or by a community. Territory is a socially constructed space linking history and economic, political, and cultural processes. Moreover, it is organized based on the relationships established by those who inhabit it, relationships that often shape it and give it meaning and identity. On the other hand, territorialization, understood as a process in which a subject, community, or social group appropriates and links itself to a physical place, opens space to debate how the relationship between subject and territory is constructed or established (Haesbaert, 2010).

Within these processes and events between individuals and the territory, there is an inherent connection between the territory and nature, which is often widely misunderstood, resulting in disconnection from communities.

The biocentric perspective of Indigenous peoples assumes that existence depends on a larger environment beyond their territory to ensure fundamental aspects, such as the sustenance of their inhabitants. The connection between the individual and the territory is a process that also requires considering the presence and participation of other species and elements of the environment. Therefore, these processes involve an emotional connection to the territory and extend beyond exclusively human activities (Krenak, 2020).

In Indigenous peoples' worldviews, a differentiation exists between space and territory. "Territory is based on space, but it is not space. It is a production from space" (Santos da Rocha, 2013, p. 139). In other words, space is a broader category than territory, highlighting the dynamic relationship between physical space and individuals.

In this logic, space is not merely a container for social interactions or waiting to be filled with human emotions; it also shapes and conditions ways of being in the world. There is a constant tension between individuals and the place, wherein individuals influence the place through their daily lives, but they are also influenced and shaped by it in return.

In this perspective, objects are not isolated from the social construction of the territory; rather, they play a crucial role in signifying, appropriating, and shaping ways of inhabiting a place.

Finally, this reading of three voices with a territorial and disciplinary perspective is an invitation to rethink our paradigms and practices to come closer to recognizing, acting, and transforming realities that we do not yet know.

The reading of these professional practices and experiences allows us to approach an understanding of these inhabited spaces where an underlying reality that is greater than the material, tangible, and physical reality coexists. It challenges us to include in our practices the constructed experiences, manifested through the historical memory of those who inhabit them.

Conclusion

On the experience with the different peoples, communities, and ethnic groups presented, a professional commitment with their roots stands out; a journey, a path is developed through territorialities, territories, and bodies through the journey, the living, and the existence of Indigenous peoples. We follow the journey and their relationships with the Kayambi, Guaraní, and Mapuche peoples to achieve an understanding of their worldview, their living, their existence, and their transcendence in an occupational therapy perspective that breaks with the coloniality of knowing and doing, with the Eurocentric technical hegemony and the proposal of a way of life disconnected from ancestry and worldview. Moreover, it is a perspective that takes actions and evaluations contextualized in the sociocultural realities of community life and an intersectional ethical-political position in the face of class, race, ethnicity, and gender relations.

References

Achig-Balarezo, D. (2019). Cosmovisión Andina. Categorias y principios. *Revista de la Facultad de Ciencias Médicas de la Universidad de Cuenca, 37*(3), 5–8. https://doi.org/10.18537/RFCM.37.03.01

Ambrosio, L., & Silva, C. R. (2022). Interseccionalidade: Um conceito amefricano e diaspórico para a terapia ocupacional. *Cadernos Brasileiros de Terapia Ocupacional, 30*, e3150.

Barros, D. D., de Almeida, M. C., & Vecchia, T. C. (2007). Terapia ocupacional social: Diversidade, cultura e saber técnico. *Revista de Terapia Ocupacional da Universidade de São Paulo, 18*(3), 128–134.

Bengoa, J. (1996) *Historia del Pueblo Mapuche (Siglos XIX y XX)* (3rd edn). Santiago de Chile: Ediciones SUR. www.sitiosur.cl/r.php?id=124

Bottinelli, M. M. (2018). ¿Por qué pensar epistemología en terapia ocupacional? In S. Simó, A. Guajardo, O. F. Correa, S. M. Galheigo, & S. García (Eds.), *Terapias Ocupacionales del Sur: Derechos Humanos, Ciudadanía y Participación* (pp. 97–113). Santiago de Chile: Editorial USACH.

Brand, A., Colman, R. S., & Machado, N. (2008). Os Guarani nas fronteiras do MERCOSUL. In *Anais da 26a Reunião Brasileira de Antropologia*, Porto Seguro, Bahia.

Chihuailaf, A. et al. (2012). *Historia y Luchas del Pueblo Mapuche*. Santiago: Editorial Aún Creemos en Los Sueños.

Chimbolema, N. A. (2017). *Estado y Cosmovisión*. https://inredh.org/archivos/pdf/c_cosmovision_2017.pdf

Churuchumbi, G. (2014). Usos cotidianos del termino Sumak Kawsay en el territorio Kayambi. Universidad Andina Simon Bolivar. https://repositorio.uasb.edu.ec/handle/10644/4055

Confederación del Pueblo Kayambi (2021). *Kintiku Yachay*. Pueblo Kayambi. https://protecciondederechoscayambe.gob.ec/wp-content/uploads/2021/06/KINTIKU-YACHAY-EDUCACI%C3%93N-PARA-LA-VIDA-COMUNITARIA.pdf

Cruz, M. (09 de Julio de 2018). Cosmovisión Andina e interculturalidad una mirada al desarrollo sostenible desde el Sumak Kawsay. *Revista Chakiñan de Ciencias Sociales y Humanidades*, (5), 119–132. http://scielo.senescyt.gob.ec/scielo.php?script=sci_serial&pid=2550-6722&lng=es&nrm=iso

Fabio, J. L. (2010). *La Salud de Los Pueblo Indígenas de las Américas*. Organización Panamericana de la Salud. paho.org/hq/dmdocuments/2009/53-SPI-conceptos-estrategias.PDF.pdf

Farinango, D. (2020). *La Participación de la Mujer en la Administración de la Justicia Indígena en el Pueblo Kayambi durante el Periodo 2015–2017*. Universidad Central del Ecuador. www.dspace.uce.edu.ec/bitstream/25000/22286/1/T-UCE-0013-JUR-290.pdf

Gálvez, M., Godoy, M., & Lagos, A. (2010). Construcción de significado de experiencia de cuerpo con personas en situación de discapacidad física adquirida. *Revista Chilena de Terapia Ocupacional*, (10), 71–83. https://doi.org/10.5354/0719-5346.2010.10562

García, S. (2014). Comprensiones de lo comunitario en Terapia Ocupacional: Aproximaciones desde la Revista Ocupación Humana, 1996–2021. *Revista Ocupación Humana, 22*(Suppl.), 102–116. https://doi.org/10.25214/25907816.1342

Giglia, A. (2012). *El Habitar y la Cultura: Perspectivas Teóricas y de Investigación*. Barcelona: Anthropos.

Glauser, M., & Villagra, R. (2020). Processos contemporâneos de despossessão e re-territorialização dos povos Ava Guarani, Mbya Guarani e Pae Tavyterã da Região Leste do Paraguai. *Revista de Estudos e Pesquisas sobre as Américas, 14*(3), 103–140.

Gonzalez, L. (2020). *Por um Feminismo Afro-Latino-Americano*. Rio de Janeiro: Zahar.

Haesbaert, R. (2010). Território e multiterritorialidade: Um debate. *GEOgraphia, 9*(17). https://doi.org/10.22409/GEOgraphia2007.v9i17.a13531

IBGE. (2010). *Os Indígenas no Censo Demográfico 2010: Primeiras Considerações com Base no Quesito Cor ou Raça*. Instituto Brasileño de Geografia y Estadística. www.ibge.gov.br/indigenas/indigena_censo2010.pdf

Krenak, A. (2020). *Ideias para Adiar o Fim do Mundo*. São Paulo: Companhia das Letras.

Ladeira, M. I., & Tupã, L. W. (2004). Condições ambientais do território guarani: Implicações no modo de vida. *Revista Tellus, 4*(6), 51–63.

Laverde, M. C. (2001). Prácticas Indígenas relacionadas con la enfermedad. *Aquichan, 1*(1), 11–13. www.scielo.org.co/scielo.php?script=sci_arttext&pid=S1657-59972001000100005

Macedo, M. D. C. (2016). *O povo Guarani da América Latina e relações interculturais nas mídias sociais virtuais: Uso e apropriação na construção de redes de cooperação*. Doctoral thesis, Federal University of Espírito Santo.

Macedo, M. D. C. et al. (2016). Olhares em formação: Refletindo a prática da terapia ocupacional em um contexto cultural a partir de experiências com povos indígenas. *Cadernos de Terapia Ocupacional da UFSCar, 24*(1), 77–89.

Macedo, M. D. C., Salamao, E. B., Figueiredo, J. L. S., & Pereira, M. Z. (2021). Autocuidado, sustentabilidade e mulheres indígenas: Do urucum à escova progressiva. *Anais do VI Seminário Nacional de Pesquisa em Terapia Ocupacional*, pp. 146–147.

Melín, M., Mansilla, P., & Royo, M. (2017). *Mapu Chillkantukun Zugu: Descolonizando el Mapa del Wallmapu, Construyendo Cartografía Cultural en Territorio Mapuche*. Temuco: Pu Lof Editories.

Milanez, F., Sá, L., Krenak, A., Cruz, F. S. M., Ramos, E. U., & Jesus, G. D. S. D. (2019). Existência e Diferença: O Racismo contra os Povos Indígenas. *Revista Direito e Práxis, 10*, 2161–2181.

Millán, S. Q., Arias-Ortega, K., Troncoso, G. M., Torres, H., et al. (2021). Conocimientos geográficos y territoriales con base epistémica en la memoria social mapuche. *Revista Brasileira de Ciências Sociais, 36*(106), e3610603.

Pino Morán, J., Ceballos Concha, M., & Sepúlveda Hernández, R. (2015). Terapia ocupacional comunitaria crítica: Dialogos y reflexiones para iniciar una propuesta colectiva. *TOG (A Coruña), 12*(22). www.revistatog.com/num22/pdfs/colab3.pdf

Pissolato, E. P. (2006). *A duração da pessoa: Mobilidade, parentesco e xamanismo mbya (Guarani)*. Doctoral thesis, National Museum of the Federal University of Rio de Janeiro.

Quintriqueo, S., Arias-Ortega, K., Muñoz, G., Morales, S., et al. (2018–2021). Sentido del lugar como conocimientos educativos territoriales mapuches para una educación intercultural (Grant No. 1181531). Fondo Nacional de Investigación Científica y Tecnológica. FONDECYT REGULAR.

Renard, J. (2009). Vanier (M.) (dir.)—Territoires, territorialité, territorialisation: Controverses et perspectives. *Norois*, (210), 109–110. https://doi.org/10.4000/norois.2770

Rengifo, G. F. (2018). *La Chakana y los Saberes Ancestrales del Pueblo Kayambi*. Universidad Central del Ecuador. www.dspace.uce.edu.ec/bitstream/25000/16876/1/T-UCE-0010-FIL-140.pdf

Rodríguez Valbuena, D. (2010). Territorio y territorialidad: Nueva categoría de análisis y desarrollo didáctico de la Geografía. *Uni-PluriVersidad, 10*(3), 90–100.

Rojas Castillo, C. P. et al. (2019). Terapia ocupacional en la ruralidad: Una experiencia en La Macarena, Meta. *Revista Ocupación Humana, 19*(2), 86–102. https://doi.org/10.25214/25907816.866

Ruiz Guerra, R., & Soriano Hernández, S. (Eds.). (2023). *Indigenismos e Indianismo en América Latina: Respuestas a la Interculturalidad*. Quadrivivium.

Santos da Rocha, A. (2013). Território como representação. *Mercator—Revista de Geografia da UFC, 12*(29), 139–153. www.redalyc.org/pdf/2736/273629350011.pdf

Silva, E. M. (2007). *Folhas ao vento: A micromobilidade de grupos Mbya e Nhandéva (Guarani) na Tríplice Fronteira*. Doctoral thesis, National Museum of the Federal University of Rio de Janeiro.

Simó, S. (2018). La teoría del renacimiento ocupacional. In S. Simó, A. Guajardo, O. F. Correa, S. M. Galheigo, & S. García (Eds.), *Terapias Ocupacionales desde el Sur: Derechos Humanos, Ciudadanía y Participación* (pp. 205–224). University of Santiago de Chile.

Simó, S., & Abregú, M. M. (2015). Ecología ocupacional: El estudio de caso de la megaminería en Argentina. *Revista Argentina de Terapia Ocupacional, 1*(25).

Teao, K. M. (2015). *Território e identidade dos Guarani Mbya do Espírito Santo (1967–2006).* Doctoral thesis, Fluminense Federal University, Niterói, RJ, Brazil.

Tubino, F. (2014). El trasfondo epistémico de los conflictos interculturales. *Contextualizaciones Latinoamericanas, 11*(7). https://contexlatin.cucsh.udg.mx/index.php/CL/article/view/2762

Yrigoyen Fajardo, R. Z. (2009). Aos 20 anos do Convênio 169 da OIT: Balanço e desafios da implementação dos direitos dos Povos Indígenas na América Latina. In R. Verdum (Ed.), *Povos Indígenas: Constituições e reformas políticas na América Latina* (pp. 9–62). Brasília: Instituto de Estudos Socioeconômicos.

Zango Martín, I. & Moruno Mirales, P. (2013). Aportaciones de la etnografía doblemente reflexiva en la construcción de la terapia ocupacional desde una perspectiva intercultural. *Revista de Antropología Iberoamericana, 8*(1), 9–48.

Zapata, J. (2010). *Espacio y territorio sagrado: Lógica del ordenamiento territorial indígena.* Post-graduate thesis, National University of Colombia. http://www.alberdi.de/ESPACIO%20%20Y%20TERRITORIO%20SAGRADO-Jair,actu,02.06.07.pdf

CHAPTER 2

Buen Vivir

COSMOVIVENCIAS FROM OCCUPATIONAL THERAPY IN DIFFERENT TERRITORIES OF ABYA YALA

Francia Elena Rocha Santos, Diana Milena Ramírez Osorio, and Erick Valdelomar Marín

Abstract

This chapter delves into the concept of *Buen Vivir*, often translated as "good living," a principle deeply rooted in the Indigenous and ancestral ways of experiencing and interpreting life in Abya Yala, the name of our territory, which the colonists called Latin America, ignoring the identity processes of our ancestors. Occupational therapy programs originated in Latin America around 1956, heavily influenced by the United States and Britain in their curricular content. This influence has conditioned the incorporation of ancestral *cosmovivencias*, ways of seeing and experiencing the world, into our professional knowledges and practices. Under this framework, the chapter raises questions: How do we recover ancestral thinking to resize the harmonic relationship between human beings, occupation, and natural context? How do we link the cosmovisions of *Buen Vivir* to rethinking our everyday lives? How can we create a respectful dialogue between ancestral knowledge and occupational therapy as a discipline? To transit through these questions, we weave intersections between the local scholarly references defining *Buen Vivir* and occupational therapies'[1] experiences situated in different territories. To conclude, the chapter proposes the analysis of a territorial experience that allows the reader to unravel the relationship between human occupation and *Buen Vivir*.

1 "Occupational therapies" refers to the multiple knowledges and practices that an occupational therapy practitioner can acquire in various contexts based on their own needs and realities. It involves the interactions between the professional, their training, the context, individuals, and collectives. We use the plural form to acknowledge that these bodies of knowledge and practices are diverse. Following this logic, ascribing a single identity to professional practice is impossible.

Keywords
Buen Vivir; occupational therapy; Abya Yala; ancestral knowledge

Learning outcomes

- Analyze the relationship between occupational therapy practices in Abya Yala territories and the *Buen Vivir* perspective.
- Discuss how the *Buen Vivir* perspective has historically interacted with and been overshadowed by colonial perspectives in Abya Yala.
- Examine the influence of Western frameworks, particularly from the United States and Britain, on the development of occupational therapy in Latin America and how these influences have affected the incorporation of ancestral *cosmovivencias* into the discipline.
- Identify ways to incorporate the *Buen Vivir* perspective into contemporary occupational therapy practices, fostering a harmonious relationship between human beings, their occupations, and their context through respectful dialogue between ancestral knowledge and contemporary occupational therapy.

Introduction

There are many nations and cultures in Abya Yala, the name of our territory, which the colonists called Latin America, ignoring the identity processes of our ancestors. Each has its own identity, but with a common essence: the community paradigm is based on living in harmony and balance with the environment. The wise men and women[2] of our ancestral peoples affirm that to recover ancestral cosmovision, we must return to our identity, a fundamental principle for knowing our origin and our complementary role in life (CAOI, 2010, p. 24).

Amongst the majority of peoples of the Andean region of Colombia, Ecuador, Bolivia, Peru, Paraguay, Chile, and Argentina, and in the ancestral peoples of Mexico, Central America, the Caribbean, and North America, the Ancestral Cosmovision or Cosmic Vision survives as a way of understanding, perceiving the world and expressing oneself in life relations (CAOI, 2010). The concept of *cosmovivencia* is understood as the essence of everyday life, uses and customs, and the relationship between human beings, their community, and their environment daily during life itself. This leads

2 Also known as *knowledgeable men and women*. Among Indigenous peoples across Abya Yala, these individuals develop the necessary abilities and sensitivity to converse with their natural surroundings and comprehend nature's messages (UNESCO, 2022).

us[3] to reflect on human thought and action in a relational key and to understand its influence on everyday actions.

Buen Vivir is a *cosmovivencia* that integrates the knowledge, beliefs, and vital practices of the original and ancestral peoples of Abya Yala; it reaffirms the defense and respect for Mother Earth, its autonomy, diversity, and cultural and spiritual identity. It also promotes the construction of social, academic, economic, and political movements as alternatives to the hegemonic development models in Abya Yala. *Buen Vivir* has acquired different symbolisms and forms of expression in the region, which is why meanings have been attributed to it in multiple languages. It is based on a life project that unifies human existence and gives meaning to what happens in everyday life (Dussel, 2009). Its philosophy has developed in different ways and has been called according to the meaning it acquires in the territories *Pura Vida*, *Vivir Bien*, *Vivir Sabroso*, and *Buen Vivir*, among others (Waldmüller, 2014).

In the Abya Yala territory, *Buen Vivir* has been recognized as a form of emancipation that highlights the organization of peoples around the survival of their knowledge, which has allowed them to maintain themselves and resist the dynamics of domination associated with different historical moments such as colonization, modernity, and modernization (Gallegos Anda, 2018; Waldmüller, 2014). Interestingly, from a Western point of view, these *cosmovivencias* are materialized in discourses such as welfare; however, ancestral knowledge has existed long before contemporary cultures and has managed to overcome historical moments. Although it is not part of this chapter to delve into the history of the processes of colonization and modernity, we recognize the importance of alluding to some moments and concepts that have impacted how we understand and appropriate the relationship between human beings and their context.

In the literature, modernity is referred to from different perspectives; Echeverría (2009) mentions that modernity can be considered as "a civilising tendency endowed with a new unitary principle of coherence or structuring for civilised social life and for the world corresponding to that life" (p. 11). In this sense, this unitary principle has implied the disregarding of other possible ways of structuring social life and imposition paradigms based on capitalism and globalization.

For Dussel (1994), modernity originated in medieval European cities when Europe confronted "The other" through complex processes of exploration and colonization spanning several centuries. Various regions' economic,

3 The collective construction of this text appropriates the expression "we" to refer to the sense of belonging of the people involved. It is assumed that we are part of the contexts, knowledge, and practices reflected here.

spiritual, and political factors influenced this confrontation. Europe defined itself as an "ego"—a discoverer, conqueror, and colonizer of the otherness that constitutes modernity itself (Contreras, 1995, p. 4). In this context, "The other" encompassed not only people from distant lands but also those from other parts of Europe, who were often portrayed as pagan, animalistic, and fit to be exploited, starved, enslaved, and conquered. This perception was shaped by historical events such as the Reconquista, the Crusades of the 1200s, and subsequent wars against pagan peoples in the Middle East and Eastern Europe. The systematic denial, stigmatization, and forced modernization of "The other" was rooted in the belief in the superiority of European culture, which regarded colonized cultures as inferior and underdeveloped. According to this logic, the violent domination exercised over the supposedly discovered "other" was seen as a profitable endeavor to "rescue them" from a backward way of life. This effort to civilize them, often by force, was presented as having an altruistic purpose, imposing new ways of thinking, being, and existing in the world. As Dussel (2020) argues, this rationale is entrenched in modernity; it presupposes the superiority of one's own culture simply because it is one's own, thereby tautologically justifying the war of conquest.

Some perspectives view modernity as an emancipatory process within the Abya Yala territory. Robles (2012) emphasizes that modernity involves the discovery of subjectivity, proposing a unique relationship between the subject and themselves, characterized by an inherent drive toward freedom achieved through reflection (p. 171). Castro-Gómez (2000) offers a critical view of modernity, describing it as "a machine that generates alterities which, in the name of reason and humanism, excludes from its imagination the hybridity, multiplicity, ambiguity, and contingency of concrete life forms" (p. 88). He further argues that postmodern philosophy and cultural studies see the current crisis of modernity as a significant historical opportunity for the emergence of long-repressed differences. Building on this perspective, Navarrete's (2019) review of Castro-Gómez's work suggests an emancipatory and political approach, anticipating the possibility of a transmodern moment. This view envisions a political project aimed at "de-Europeanizing" the legacy of modernity, potentially allowing for a more inclusive and diverse understanding of social and cultural realities.

For example, in the Andean region, *Buen Vivir* or *Sumay Kawsay* (in Quechua) represents the reclamation of the essence of historically repressed cultures, which embrace spirituality and care for oneself, others, and nature as fundamental principles. In this context, collective thought is prioritized over individual thought, and existence is constructed from these interconnected relationships. The cosmovisions of our ancestral peoples, related to

Buen Vivir, precede the concept of well-being that arose in European contexts, despite claims that this well-being emerged as a response to the adverse effects of exploitation, domination, and consumerism (CIDI, 2021).

Another viewpoint is related to *Vivir Sabroso*, which is part of the Afrocentric linguistic heritage of the Pacific communities in Chocó, Colombia. Its philosophy is rooted in a long tradition of life that dialogues with African philosophies such as *Ubuntu* and *Muntu* (Copete, Lozano, & Valencia, 2020; Lozano & Copete, 2019). *Ubuntu* develops principles of interconnectedness with other people, creating possibilities to build and create together based on recognizing interdependence as a foundation for well-being. This philosophy emphasizes the necessity of recognizing the presence and tangible existence of others. In contrast, *Muntu* is a holistic concept representing an integral vision of the universe from various African cultures, particularly the Bantu. It encompasses human, natural, astral, and divine beings interwoven in a continuum that unites past, present, and future (Copete et al., 2020, p. 25). This perspective highlights the importance of understanding the self as part of a space, a time, and a community. It challenges the individualism imposed by modern and "developed" cultures, where the emphasis on personal independence has led people to view themselves as self-sufficient, resulting in alienation and negative impacts on their physical and mental health.

This reflection is important for the development of occupational therapies because, in the hegemonic practices of the field, a person's independence is often measured by their level of functionality and capacity. This approach neglects the impact of the ability to relate and co-construct with others and the natural world on human development. It is necessary to consider these issues to understand how occupational therapies' knowledge, practices, and resistance have evolved in Abya Yala. Recognizing that the traditional knowledge of the profession has been shaped by Eurocentric models, which prioritize a hegemonic clinical view of the discipline with an emphasis on the individual and hierarchical relationships in knowledge, practices, and people, is a crucial starting point.

As an act of resistance, occupational therapies in Abya Yala have shifted from clinical spaces to understanding occupational needs in social and community contexts, such as the home, school, workplace, and natural environments like forests, rivers, waterfalls, and springs. This shift has highlighted the importance of the collective as a constituent of being. It has allowed for the interpretation of realities in everyday life and the territories where people interact and find meaning in their lives. Recognizing the inseparable relationship between doing and the natural world, this approach emphasizes the importance of the collective in constituting being and interpreting realities through these interactions.

Prioritizing encounters with people in their daily lives, respecting their natural, ancestral, relational, and binding context, and assuming co-construction as a principle requires occupational therapies to establish a transversal dialogue between the different ways of being, doing, and living. This practice has been called "emergent." This chapter proposes a transition between the constructs of *Buen Vivir* and the notions of territory, interculturality, spirituality, and critical thinking as a basis for understanding the link between *Buen Vivir* and occupational therapies.

Bringing the *Buen Vivir* approach to occupational therapy in the territories of Abya Yala

The invention of development as a global model for economic and technological progress has brought the world to the brink of a vital social, economic, ecological, and political crisis (Escobar, 2014). There is an urgent need for everyone to understand and incorporate other worldviews that allow us to value our natural environment, our connections with nature, ourselves, and the people around us. It is essential to think collectively, prioritize ancestral knowledge and practices, and recognize that we are interdependent and everything is connected. In this context, *Buen Vivir* is more than a concept; it reflects the *cosmovivencia* of the peoples of Abya Yala. *Buen Vivir* embodies the essence of everyday life, customs, and the relationships between human beings, their community, and their environment. In other words, it represents everyday life. This idea has been increasingly reflected in and appropriated by occupational therapies in Abya Yala.

While occupational therapies' practices in community contexts are a reality, they have often been shaped by hegemonic perspectives related to concepts such as public health and well-being, as reflected in government policies, health corporations, and hierarchies within medicine and healthcare. Thus, there is a lack of an integrated approach that weaves the principles of *Buen Vivir* into the discipline's work. Despite this, academic efforts have been made to link the cosmovisions of *Buen Vivir* to training practices. For example, the University of Guayaquil, in 2018, constructed its academic plan based on the Ecuadorian government's ten-year plan,[4] which integrated the perspective of *Buen Vivir* (Vélez, 2022). This shift in perspective represented a move toward recognizing Indigenous knowledge and sustainable living practices in national development. Although this initiative resonated

4 The Ten Year Education Plan of Ecuador, projected from 2006 to 2015 by the Ecuadorian Ministry of Education, aimed to respond to the population's needs through a comprehensive state management strategy. This plan sought to stabilize and organize various priorities with an inclusive, multicultural, and multi-ethnic approach.

with the political context at the time, emphasizing social and environmental well-being over purely economic growth, it has since undergone changes that have sidelined this perspective (Vélez, 2022).

The following section will explore the constructs of Abya Yala and *Buen Vivir* that are essential for the proposed reflection and the implementation of occupational therapy.

Essence and constructs of Abya Yala and *Buen Vivir*

According to Arias (2017), Abya Yala represents the Latin American continent from an Indigenous perspective. *Abya* means "blood," symbolizing life among Mesoamerican peoples, and *yala* means "mountain" (Arias, 2017, p. 2). In the language of the Kuna people, *abya yala* means "ripe land," "living land," or "flourishing land," synonymous with America. The Kuna people originated in northern Colombia's Sierra Nevada, inhabited the Gulf of Urabá and the Darien Mountains, and now live on the coast of Panama in the Kuna Yala comarca (Porto-Gonçalves & Rego-Monteiro, 2022). According to Arias (2020), the first recorded use of Abya Yala instead of "America" can be traced back to 1507, when it appeared in the work of German cosmographer Martin Waldseemüller (1475–1522). However, it was consecrated in the late 18th and early 19th centuries and used during Latin American independence movements, mainly due to its adoption by Criollo elites—individuals of European descent born in the Americas who held significant power in colonial society. These elites, seeking to distinguish themselves from their European counterparts, embraced Abya Yala as a symbolic rejection of colonial names and a reclamation of Indigenous terminology. This choice reflected their complex position: asserting a uniquely American identity while maintaining their privileged status. Abya Yala thus became a tool for Criollo elites to navigate the tension between their European heritage and American birth, embodying their desire to forge a distinct identity separate from European influence (Escobar, 2016).

The term "Latin America" emerged after modernity/coloniality, whereas Abya Yala represents the opposite: the territory's precolonial and ancestral identity. It acknowledges the ancestral names of mountains, rivers, plants, animals, and everything surrounding us, making the space our own. This imbues it with meanings and recognizes it as territories laden with struggles, ancestral memories, and the essence of freedom. It indicates that it is not merely a name but a political statement, emphasizing the importance of recognizing ourselves as part of Abya Yala.

Embracing the concept of Abya Yala involves reconnecting with life, nature, and the delicate balance between humans, plants, and animals. This perspective, rooted in ancestral Indigenous Andean philosophies such as *Buen Vivir* (Spanish), *Sumak Kawsay* (Quechua), and *Suma Qamaña* (Aymara), emphasizes our role as part of a larger community rather than isolated individuals. These philosophies, each with distinct origins and nuances, oppose the Western view that prioritizes economic growth and development at the expense of *Allpamama* (Mother Earth). The Western approach often alienates humans from life's essence, reducing them to mere producers or consumers detached from natural rhythms. The concept of Abya Yala extends beyond Indigenous communities, encompassing the diaspora of Afro-descendent communities and mestizos who claim their ancestry without direct Indigenous or African roots (Arias, 2017). While many Latin Americans have mixed heritage that may include both Indigenous and African influences to varying degrees, it is crucial to recognize the distinct nature of these philosophies. Each reflects the unique experiences and worldviews of specific communities, and conflating them would oversimplify their rich cultural diversity.

Central to this analysis are the 13 principles of the Andean cosmovision described by Fernando Huanacuni Mamani in a text published by the Andean Coordination of Indigenous Organizations (CAOI, 2010). These principles are:

- Knowing how to eat.
- Knowing how to drink.
- Knowing how to dance.
- Knowing how to sleep.
- Knowing how to work.
- Knowing how to meditate.
- Knowing how to think.
- Knowing how to love and be loved.
- Knowing how to listen.
- Knowing how to speak well.
- Knowing how to dream.
- Knowing how to walk.
- Knowing how to give and receive.

The following section will describe the elements of *Buen Vivir* and their interaction with occupational therapy professional practices.

Reflect

Choose one of the 13 principles of the Andean cosmovision that resonates with you. Write briefly about:

- How do you currently practice this principle from your own worldview?
- How can you incorporate it more intentionally into your life?

Elements from *Buen Vivir* that interact with occupational therapy practice

Buen Vivir and territory

The conceptions surrounding the notion of territory are varied and multifaceted. Territory can be understood as a physical space, a place of exchange and production, a site for social events, or a relational space where senses and meanings are intertwined, reflecting social complexity. For Indigenous peoples, territory embodies numerous meanings tied to their worldview, emphasizing the interwoven existential relationship between humans and nature. This relationship is seen as mutually beneficial, protective, and preservative (CAOI, 2010).

From a social perspective, territory is linked to community, serving as a meeting place where common cultures and histories are interwoven. It is a material and symbolic space for relationships and interactions that can foster social cohesion (Ramírez et al., 2022). These interactions create social practices that generate complementarity, reciprocity, or confrontation relationships. These dynamics constantly evolve, leading to an understanding of territory as a cultural construction (Capel, 2016). The territory as a reality in which actors with different interests relate to each other in confluences, tensions, disputes, and resistances makes visible professional undertakings that seek to recognize the local social dynamics, the singular experiences of subjects and/or collectives, and the links they establish in everyday actions. It would seem that looking at these aspects invites us to assume more collective and horizontal forms of construction in the territories among the different actors (Ramírez et al., 2022).

The countries of the Abya Yala territory have long faced challenges related to political and collective conceptions of territory. These struggles often represent efforts to defend and reclaim subjectivities and freedoms. Escobar (2014) notes that the perseverance of communities and ethnic-territorial grassroots movements involves resistance, opposition, defense, and affirmation of their territories.

Think and Discuss

The reflection in this text aims to analyze the dynamics through which local understandings and knowledge are constructed and their global applicability. Consider and discuss the following questions:

- Is a universal conception of knowledge always possible?
- What are the consequences of assuming global knowledge as the basis for local practices?
- Can local knowledge be transferred and applied universally?
- Which local knowledge and practices are valued for their global potential?

These questions will help us explore the balance between global and local knowledge and the importance of recognizing and valuing diverse ways of knowing.

Occupational therapy focuses on the senses and meanings attributed to the activities individuals or groups choose and perform and their significance to their lives. Humans are inherently occupational beings, and their participation in occupations occurs in spaces where they relate to others. In this context, occupation has a sociocultural function, is systemic, and occurs within a specific territory defined by space and time (Rojas, 2011).

Reflecting on occupational therapy practices through the lens of territory as a relational space encourages us to consider the places where these therapies occur. We propose an analysis of these spaces, both outwardly and inwardly. In our practices, we identify the physical spaces where the communities, families, and individuals we work with are situated (outward analysis). Additionally, it is crucial to consider the spaces occupied by occupational therapists and their interactions with *Buen Vivir*'s worldviews (inward analysis).

We could differentiate between *Buen Vivir* in professional practices in traditional and so-called "emerging" contexts. An example could be the reflection on the usual location of occupational therapy services, often with limited physical space and resources for professional practice with dignity. They are often assigned spaces such as under the stairs in a school, the attic in a hospital, or the smallest space in a community center. From the geopolitics of actions, we must ask: What impact does the spatial location of occupational therapy services have on interdisciplinary teams and service users? Professionals frequently struggle to assert and highlight the importance of their care.

Another example pertains to the scenarios of professional work established by academia, which often prioritize institutional practices while overlooking community contexts. This raises the question: Does clinical reasoning apply to everyday contexts, or should we adopt professional reasoning that embraces diverse spaces? The traditional association of occupational therapy with biomedical models can hinder the profession's positioning in labor, educational, and community settings. Consequently, employers' demands often do not align with the occupational therapist's professional profile needed to address community needs. Thus, the involvement of occupational therapists in extramural, community, and everyday scenarios results from political advocacy and the persistent assertion of their knowledge and practices. This positions occupational therapy practice in Abya Yala as a collective and political endeavor.

These "other" spaces[5] are often described as emerging in academic discourse. However, in the Abya Yala territories, they are integral to everyday life and natural professional actions, reflecting their unique realities. Therefore, it is logical for actions aimed at enhancing the occupational participation of individuals or groups within their everyday environments. This raises important questions: From whose perspective are these everyday life scenarios considered emerging? For whom do these non-clinical scenarios emerge?

Another example concerns the scenarios of professional work established by academia, which often serves as the authority on professional practice. This framework frequently recognizes practices as institutional and becomes less defined in other contexts, such as community settings. Does clinical reasoning apply to everyday contexts, or should we adopt professional reasoning that embraces diverse spaces? The traditional association of occupational therapy with biomedical models can hinder the profession's positioning in work-based, educational, and community settings. As a result, employers' demands often do not align with the occupational therapist's professional profile needed to address community needs. Additionally, it can be affirmed that the linking of occupational therapists to extramural, community, and everyday scenarios has been the result of political advocacy and the constant

5 That is, different from institutional or intramural spaces, such as clinics, hospitals, health centers.

vindication of their knowledge and practices by professionals, which could situate the practice of occupational therapies in Abya Yala as a collective and political practice.

Occupational performance, a key focus in occupational therapy, emerges from the complex interplay of individuals' beliefs, values, preferences, and opportunities within their social contexts. In Abya Yala's territories, social inequality's impact on participation in occupations is undeniable. Traditional professional practices often confine interactions to institutional settings, resulting in totalizing[6] spaces with highly regulated dynamics with *others* we "attend to" or "accompany." However, adopting a *Buen Vivir* perspective could transform occupational therapy practices. This approach encourages therapists to engage in diverse spaces beyond institutional boundaries, fostering a deeper understanding of social realities. By doing so, therapists can establish meaningful connections with those they accompany, recognizing social realities and leading to mutual learning, re-signification, and transformation of professional practice.

As a result of complex social, cultural, and political struggles that have intensified over the past decade, some of the Abya Yala territories have been pioneers in the appropriation of the cosmovisions proposed by *Buen Vivir* into their political and social structures, as is the case of Ecuador and Bolivia, by including in their constitutions sanctioned in 2008 a new notion of development centered on the concept of *Sumak Kawsay* (in Quechua), *Suma Qamaña* (in Aymara), or *Buen Vivir* (in Spanish) and the right of nature, which implies a conceptual rupture (Escobar, 2014, p. 30).

These structural struggles cannot be separated from professional practice. The tendency is to integrate these worldviews into our training and professional practices to understand, reflect on, and transform the occupational participation of individuals or collectives. However, if we position ourselves as occupational therapists, we must ask ourselves: To what extent do we truly connect with people and communities in their territories? Do we have their consent to enter their realities? Do we appreciate the opportunity to be there? Do we offer our knowledge without assuming it to be the absolute truth? These questions highlight practices related to *Buen Vivir*, as they involve recognizing others, maintaining balance with the environment, and understanding professional practice from a relational logic based on respect and collective construction.

In conclusion, reflecting on our professional practice through the lenses

6 A totalizing space is referred to as one that unifies people, homogenizes them, and in that sense, standardizes forms of care and "therapies" given by evidence as effective, according to protocols and care guidelines.

of territory and *Buen Vivir* becomes an affirmative political action. It enables us to recognize, rethink, adapt, re-signify, and transform ourselves continuously (Bianchi & Serrata, 2021).

Buen Vivir and interculturality in occupational therapy

Interculturality, from the perspective of *Buen Vivir*, is not about a juxtaposition or mixture of cultures but rather an encounter between cultures. It recognizes that Eurocentric and Western knowledge has historically been placed on a plane of superiority (Gudynas & Acosta, 2011). From the perspective of *Buen Vivir*, interculturality acknowledges that all cultures possess valuable knowledge and rejects the imposition of any single culture as dominant. Ancestral peoples such as the Araona, Aymaras, Quechua, Ashuar, Kichwa of Pastaza, Kuna, Tzeltal of Chiapas, Kolla, Guaraníes, Mapuches, Bribrís, Cabecar, and Malekus across the territories of Abya Yala—Ecuador, Bolivia, Mexico, Colombia, Paraguay, Argentina, Panama, and Costa Rica—embrace *Buen Vivir* as a way of life, where relational, biocentric, ecosophical, and communal aspects prevail.

However, Moya (2009) points out that interculturality has not been uniformly developed or assimilated. The worldview of Latin America's Indigenous peoples has historically been colonized and continues to be affected by globalization and prevailing economic models. From a critical and reflexive occupational therapy perspective, there is a desire to move away from understanding interculturality through a Western or Eurocentric lens (Sarango, 2010). The Ecuadorian Indigenous leader and rector of the Amawtay Wasi University of Ecuador describes Western interculturality as characterized by:

- *Subordinate interculturality*: Indigenous peoples have experienced this over the last 500 years, where a colonial difference between cultures, Indigenous and non-Indigenous, is established.
- *Institutionalized interculturality*: Established at the level of laws as respect for differences but not respected in practice, reflecting the double discourse of modernity.
- *Intercultural folklore*: Promoted in commercial contexts, exoticizing and using features of native cultures to add value to goods and services, such as costumes, cuisine, and languages.

Occupational therapy from the *Buen Vivir* approach should aim to understand interculturality as "a new form of citizen coexistence, in diversity and harmony with nature, to achieve good living, the *Sumak Kawsay*" (Tribunal Constitucional del Ecuador, Asamblea Constituyente, 2008, p. 3). This approach involves creating a society that respects the dignity of individuals and communities in all dimensions. This perspective, affirmed by the Constituent Assembly of Ecuador, is echoed by Sarango (2010), who advocates for interculturality with equity and reciprocity.

In this manner, *Buen Vivir* can complement, guide, and transform the positioning and practices of occupational therapy regarding diversity and culture. It envisions these aspects beyond a person-centered approach to the profession, oriented toward service delivery and fostering an inclusive society where people benefit from equitable opportunities for participation, as indicated by the WFOT (2010). This perspective includes understanding interculturality concerning the natural world, as conceived by *Buen Vivir*'s worldview of the original peoples of Abya Yala.

Therefore, the perspective on diversity and culture proposed in the WFOT (2010) position statement for occupational therapists could be rethought from the perspective of *Buen Vivir*. This would allow for a more comprehensive integration of interculturality and human diversity, as shown in Table 2.1. *Buen Vivir*'s unique approach links diversity with the natural world, considers everyday experiences as evidence, and promotes respect and relational perspectives.

Table 2.1 Rethinking WFOT's position statement on diversity and culture from *Buen Vivir*'s perspective of interculturality

WFOT position statement	*Buen Vivir*'s perspective of interculturality
Diversity matters: evidence from research	Diversity matters from the ancestral cosmovision of *Buen Vivir*. *Buen Vivir* links diversity with the natural world of Abya Yala and considers people's everyday experiences in their contexts as evidence.
Human rights and inclusion matter: occupation, participation, cultural awareness and sensitivity	The *Buen Vivir* encompasses the rights of the natural world of Abya Yala and, from a relational perspective, the link between the natural world and the human world as constitutive of meaning and significance.
Language matters: the power of words	*Buen Vivir* has the conscious practice of trying to take care of our words and what is put on the table when we engage with people in their communal being from the different modes of interaction. It understands that communities' individual and collective realities are relevant to assertive communication.
Competence matters: attitude, knowledge, and skills	*Buen Vivir* promotes respect as a core competence, encouraging the conscious involvement of the natural world (Abya Yala) in occupational therapy accompaniment based on understanding different worldviews. It views competencies as opportunities to transform individual attitudes into collective well-being.

Diversity is a transversal axis for occupational therapies, which understands that each being is unique, as is their relationship with meaningful occupations. In the same way, it is understood that the relationship with the natural world through participation in occupations is singular. From the perspective of *Buen Vivir*, the extension of rights to the natural world (Abya Yala) and the recognition of how essential they are allows, in turn, for the recognition of ancestral forms of construction of meaning and significance inherent to the practices of occupational therapies that promote participation in meaningful occupations for individuals and collectives.

Recognizing the value of language and the power of words for occupational therapy practices is an opportunity to become aware of the power of what we communicate from our role in society. What we communicate can favor the recognition of diversity, capacities, resources, and possibilities, or, on the contrary, it can generate greater stigma, deprivation, or exclusion.

Buen Vivir can contribute to the acquisition of professional competencies aimed at facilitating the *development of attitudes, knowledge, and skills* of respect and recognition of the other, which allow us to understand the importance of consciously involving the natural world (Abya Yala) in the processes of occupational therapy accompaniment and moving toward collective well-being. This can be related to the following:

> Confronting development—not routinely accepting it as the panacea of paragraph IV proposed by President Harry Truman in 1949—is vital for us in the dependent world. It is vital because in it are played the autonomy, the personality and the culture, the productive bases, and the vision of the world that have given us the breath of life as human beings and peoples worthy of respect and of a better future. (Fals Borda, 2014, p. 43)

The collective action of social movements is once again important as an essential part of the awakening through popular struggle. To this end, in the Third World,[7] we have an inexhaustible diversity of cultures and peoples and exuberant tropical biodiversity, which constitute key political, social, and natural facts for our defense in the face of violent, creeping, and greedy global capitalist exploitation (Escobar, 2014, p. 42). Cultural diversity is thus ratified as a transforming force insofar as it allows for the recognition of others and the overcoming of the individuality imposed by the models of development and modernity.

7 The term "Third World" is related to the Global South. It is a concept that cannot be understood without considering global capitalism and the rise of global hierarchies and inequalities that it produced (Sajed, 2020).

Good living and spirituality

For our peoples, spirituality is a fundamental component of personal, family, and community development. It is not something detached from daily life or related to attending a specific place on a certain day or reading particular books. Instead, many cultural practices, such as dance, music, interaction with the land (*chakra*), life, and nature, are accompanied by spiritual and ancestral strength. One could say that spirituality and these practices are inseparable. For instance, asking permission to use a plant for healing purposes is a respectful practice, considering that the plant also has a spirit, as does everything around it.

Discussing spirituality from the perspective of occupational therapy leads us to recognize its vital role in everyday practice. It is understood that spirituality is not merely religious but transcends religious affiliation or rituals. It encompasses all possible ways of connecting with oneself and a dimension beyond earthly possibilities, inviting a connection with aspects unknown to science (Santacruz, 2002).

Due to its complexity, spirituality has been viewed from various perspectives in conceptual occupational therapy models. For example, in the Canadian Model of Occupational Performance, spirituality is seen as an all-pervasive life force, the manifestation of a higher reality, the source of will and self-determination, and the perception of meaning, purpose, and connection that people experience in the context of their environment (Egan, 1997).

For authors such as Iwama and Simó (2008), the concept of spirituality is closely related to the Kawa Model, which uses the Japanese term *mizu* (water) to represent functions and meanings such as fluidity, purity, spirit, cleanliness, and renewal. By coining the metaphor of the river, water is used to represent a person's energy or vital flow. Other authors have also highlighted this important aspect of life. For example, Da Silva Araújo, Da Silva Oliveira, and Rolack (2014) state that spirituality is recognized and valued "as an element capable of enhancing the meaning of occupations and directly influencing the occupational performance of clients" (p. 2). In a broader sense, we consider the concept of spirituality proposed by Bellingham et al. (1989) as three interconnected spheres: connection with oneself, connection with others, and connection with the rest of creation.

Spirituality is considered an integral part of occupational therapy practice, as any occupation or activity that holds meaning and allows an individual to achieve fulfillment in daily life involves a spiritual experience. It is important to clarify that spirituality, in this context, should not be confused with religion. While it can include religious activities and expressions, spirituality encompasses a broader range of experiences (Da Silva Araújo et al., 2014). From the perspective of *Buen Vivir* in an occupational context, sociologist Adriana Rodríguez Salazar describes spirituality as the essence of good living (Rodríguez, 2016). It is the message that ancestors left written in the clouds, the stones, and the hearts of all beings inhabiting the planet. Now is the time to return to our origins, remember who we are, and embrace the concept of *ser estando y estar siendo* (interpreted as being in both space and self or as being while present) as expressed in the Andes and the jungle.

Good living and critical thinking in occupational therapy

The conceptual and philosophical foundations of Latin American occupational therapies began to develop more than 60 years ago. As Gómez Lillo and Imperatore Blanche (2021) note, the theoretical and philosophical foundations initially developed in the United States and Britain started to evolve and transform in different countries over time, adapting to the particularities of their contexts and realities. Therefore, as Martín-Baró (1972) suggests, Latin American occupational therapists must recognize that adopting transcultural and transhistorical models created under different circumstances can significantly distort our people and our problems.

Consequently, the relationship of occupational therapy practice to *hegemonic and dominant models* must be acknowledged (Guajardo, 2016). As Kuhn (1971) states, ideology and paradigms permeate us all, conditioning our ways of thinking, acting, and relating to the world, society, and others. This directly influences the ontological conception of human beings, Mother Earth, and human occupation, potentially limiting the professional practices of occupational therapists with Indigenous populations.

Thus, to co-construct from the *Buen Vivir* worldview, occupational therapists must initially understand that Latin American countries, as Álvarez and González (2018) mention, are characterized by diverse cultural, social, political, and economic developments. These developments partly stem from the Indigenous groups that first inhabited these territories and their reactions to colonizing practices. They also share issues that shape our societies and exacerbate inequalities and exclusion, such as colonization, military dictatorships, wars, corruption and poverty, drug trafficking, migration, globalization, political and economic system changes, neoliberalism, and free trade agreements.

Another crucial element in transforming the critical thinking of occupational therapies from the *Buen Vivir* perspective is recognizing the historical exclusion and lack of participation of Indigenous populations in their well-being processes. These populations must participate in decision-making and problem-solving within their communities and territories. When occupational therapists are unaware of this reality, as Martín-Baró (1972) describes, they may align their professional practices with the "official ideology," subjecting social groups to a dominant discourse that denies, ignores, or disguises essential aspects of reality, naturalizing inequalities, and stigmas (MNICR, 2017).

Furthermore, understanding that *Indigenous peoples, Mother Earth, her natural resources and biodiversity, and the universe have a holistic and inseparable relationship that sustains their concept of life* (MNICR, 2017) is central to transforming thought and action. Recognizing and understanding the development of Indigenous cultural systems—knowledge, norms of life, production systems and Indigenous economy, conservation, access and use of resources—through which they obtain food, medicine, raw materials, handicrafts, and economic resources, practice their customs and traditions, and achieve food sovereignty and good living, is fundamental for generating critical thinking on how occupational therapists should co-construct with communities from an ecology of knowledge that develops horizontally. In order to do so, Guajardo (2016) proposes that we must free ourselves from dominant institutional discourse and practices, moving toward occupational therapies that transcend established margins and understand the millenary social struggles of our native peoples. This shift questions the paradigmatic bias and highlights the contradictions between dominant ideological approaches, theories, and models and the real needs of people and territories regarding health, education, culture, employment, and citizen participation (Vindas-Acosta & Valdelomar-Marín, 2021).

In reality, Indigenous peoples do not typically recognize occupational therapy as a natural ally in their social struggles (Guajardo, 2016), as our practice is often viewed through the lens of science, specifically occupational science, which can lead to a perception that it overlooks the needs, spirituality, worldview, beliefs, values, and meanings of Indigenous communities. This perception can be changed by acknowledging that we are historical products of these communities and that their worldview, based on *Buen Vivir*, can enhance the coexistence of all people in their permanent and inseparable relationship with Mother Earth—a relationship rooted in everyday activities.

In this sense, *Buen Vivir* should be understood, as Marques and Roldan (2020) share, as a set of ideas, knowledge, and practices that constitute an alternative to the development model in Latin America. *Buen Vivir* should be seen as an open model not exclusive to Indigenous peoples and that can be combined with other ontologies. The essential point, as Rivera Cusicanqui (2011) indicates, is to understand that the preservation of the commons is the responsibility of all and that harmony between living beings, both human and non-human, and the construction of alternative forms of sustenance are only possible under egalitarian conditions.

Latin American critical occupational therapy, as referred to by Pino and Ulloa (2016), embraces the concept of "decolonizing human occupation." This means understanding occupation as a diverse historical expression, a praxis in constant transformation, and a human potential that evolves through social tensions and struggles, paradigm shifts, and the development of productive forces within communities (Pino & Ulloa, 2016, p. 426). This perspective is vital for working collaboratively with Indigenous populations. Critical thinking calls for a break from traditional occupational therapy practices, enabling us to build with communities and promote autonomy and citizenship based on recognizing the community as an active subject and producer of its reality (Guajardo, 2016).

As an alternative model of development from the Indigenous peoples of Abya Yala, *Buen Vivir* should prompt us to question the meaning of our daily practice and its political, ethical, and aesthetic implications, as Moruno and Talavera (2007) suggest. This involves considering the subjects we address and understanding ourselves within a specific time and place. We must gain sufficient perspective to identify the influences that have shaped and continue to shape our professional work today and the consequences of our actions (Moruno & Talavera, 2007).

Critical thinking in occupational therapy challenges the imposed notions of development that overlook other ways of constructing knowledge. It recognizes that the collective action of social movements can lead to significant awakening through popular struggle. *Buen Vivir* represents a model of ancestral critical thinking that resists dominant socioeconomic models, advocating for a collective consciousness of well-being that encompasses social and natural environments rather than focusing solely on individual well-being.

Reflective Exercise: Situated Experience of *Buen Vivir*

This reflective exercise is based on a life experience described by the authors to explore the link between *Buen Vivir* and occupational therapy practice.

Josefina and Rigoberto live in the Abya Yala territory and belong to an Indigenous community where different ancestral peoples converge: Indigenous, peasant, and Afro-descendent communities. For more than four decades, these populations have faced numerous challenges, including:

- Land tenure struggles.
- Cultural, ethnic, and racial differences.

- Lack of access to basic health services, education, housing, culture, recreation, and sports.
- Non-prioritization of government intervention in their territories.
- Stigmatization of their ancestral knowledge and practices.
- Lack of social investment for the development of their territories.
- Unmet basic needs (clothing, food, housing).
- Lack of opportunities for economic well-being.
- Exploitation of natural resources and lack of conservation efforts, leading to issues such as sexual exploitation, job insecurity, and forced displacement.
- Presence of illegal armed groups, resulting in forced disappearances, violence, displacement, substance abuse, involvement of children and adolescents in armed groups, family breakdown, and mental health problems.

Josefina, 43, and Rigoberto, 56, are parents of five children: two daughters and three sons, one of whom has an intellectual disability. Originally from a peasant territory far from Josefina's, Rigoberto joined the Indigenous community more than 25 years ago, where he met Josefina. He has been a social leader, fighting for territorial rights and recognizing Indigenous knowledge. He is an empirical educator who has worked as a teacher in his community.

Josefina, native to the Indigenous community, has never had access to formal education. She learned weaving, herbal remedies, and traditional midwifery from her mother and grandmother. She manages the household, cares for the children, and works in the *chakra*.

Their eldest son, Pedro, 24, was recruited by the army at 18 and spent two years in military service due to not finishing high school. He found this experience traumatic and chose not to return to his village, migrating to the city for work and education.

Their second daughter, Juana, 19, was a survivor of sexual abuse at 13 when an oil construction site was established in their territory; the perpetrators remain unknown.

Their third son, Jojanes, 17, has an intellectual disability caused by exposure to toxic agrochemicals used by the national government to fumigate illicit crops during Josefina's pregnancy.

In 2007, due to threats and Rigoberto's forced disappearance, Josefina, pregnant at the time, had to migrate with her children to the nearest town. Speaking only her native language, she sold her weavings on the streets, where she met a woman from an NGO supporting women heads of households. This connection led to psychosocial support from an interdisciplinary team that included an occupational therapist.

For reflection

Considering the above story and the commitments to *Buen Vivir* and occupational therapy, explore how an accompaniment process can be generated from occupational therapy.

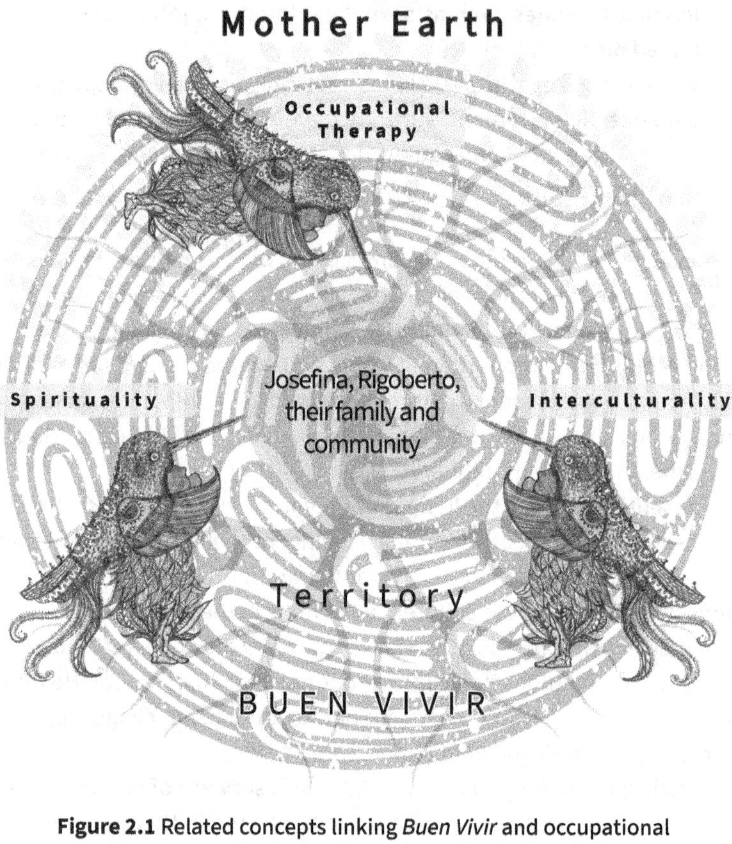

Figure 2.1 Related concepts linking *Buen Vivir* and occupational therapy practice in the Abya Yala territories (made by Pamela Talero based on drafts by the authors)

Figure 2.1 proposes a structure that correlates the aspects developed in the chapter, serving as a basis for reflection. Review Figure 2.1, which illustrates the interconnectedness of interculturality, spirituality, and occupational therapy centered around Josefina, Rigoberto, their family, and their community within a territory embedded in Mother Earth.

Reflect on the following questions and write down your thoughts:

Interculturality:

- How can occupational therapy practices honor and integrate the diverse cultural backgrounds and ancestral knowledge of Josefina and Rigoberto's community?
- What strategies can be implemented to foster intercultural dialogue and collaboration within the community?

Spirituality:

- In what ways does spirituality shape the daily occupations and well-being of Josefina and Rigoberto's family?
- How can occupational therapy incorporate spiritual practices and beliefs to enhance healing and promote harmony with nature?

Occupational therapy:

- How can occupational therapy address the family's holistic needs (physical, mental, social, and spiritual) while respecting their cultural context and connection to the land?
- What interventions can be co-created with the community to support meaningful occupations that align with their values and relationship to Mother Earth?

Territory:

- How does the community's relationship with their territory and Mother Earth influence their occupations and *Buen Vivir*?
- What role can occupational therapy play in supporting the community's efforts to protect and preserve their ancestral lands?
- How can occupational interventions be designed to strengthen the community's connection to their territory and promote sustainable practices?

Develop an action plan. Based on your reflections, outline a comprehensive action plan for how you, as an occupational therapist, would work with Josefina, Rigoberto, and their community from a *Buen Vivir* perspective. Consider the following:

- How will you engage with the community in a culturally respectful manner?

- What steps will you take to learn about and incorporate the community's ancestral knowledge and practices?
- How will you address the specific needs of Josefina, Rigoberto, and their children while considering the broader community context?
- What strategies will you employ to promote collective well-being and strengthen the community's connection to their territory?
- How will you ensure that your interventions are sustainable and aligned with the principles of *Buen Vivir*?

Note: If you are in a classroom or workshop setting, form small groups to discuss your action plans. Share insights and strategies and consider how different approaches might be integrated for a more effective practice. Each group will present their action plan to the larger group, highlighting key strategies and expected outcomes. Be prepared to provide feedback and suggestions to your peers, focusing on how well the plans incorporate the principles of *Buen Vivir* and respect for Mother Earth.

Conclusions

- From *Buen Vivir*'s perspective, it is essential to understand that occupational therapy practice must be immersed in the contexts in which people and groups live their daily lives. This approach is crucial for accessing the diverse meanings necessary for collaboratively designing accompaniment processes.

- Based on the narrative and methodological proposal at the end of this text, we position occupational therapy from a perspective different from the colonial one, which often regards professions, their knowledge, and practices as hegemonic and dominant. The potential for generating synergies and transformations in the social realities of the people and groups we accompany depends on our ability to co-construct viable alternatives that promote harmony and good living.

- Thinking of occupational therapy in terms of *Buen Vivir* involves shifting from an individual to a collective consciousness, recognizing the interconnection between people and the natural world. It allows us to affirm that participation in occupations results from collective action; people are inherently occupational and interdependent by nature.

- Using expressions in our discourse that integrate us into the contexts and social dynamics we accompany can foster relationships of closeness and meaning. This, in turn, can influence our knowledge and professional practices, making them more flexible and serving people and communities.

References

Álvarez, J. L., & González, M. (2018). La ocupación como derecho: Reflexiones del 33er Consejo y 17° Congreso Mundial de la Federación Mundial de Terapeutas Ocupacionales. *Revista de la Ocupación Humana, 18*(1), 3–6.

Arias, A. (2017). Indigenous knowledges and sites of Indigenous memory. *TRANSMODERNITY: Journal of Peripheral Cultural Production of the Luso-Hispanic World*, 7(1), 1–17.

Arias, A. (2020). Reconfigurando mundos, combatiendo el pensamiento eurocéntrico: Los desafíos planteados por las narrativas indígenas del continente. *Revista Iberoamericana, 36*(272), 683–698.

Bellingham, R., Cohen, B., Jones, T., & Spaniol, L. (1989). Connectedness: Some skills for spiritual health. *American Journal of Health Promotion, 4*(1), 18–31.

Bianchi, P. C., & Serrata, M. A. (2021). Anotaciones sobre conceptos y prácticas de territorio y comunidad en la Terapia Ocupacional colombiana. *Ocupación Humana*, 6–26. https://doi.org/10.25214/25907816.1066

CAOI. (2010, June). *Buen Vivir/Vivir Bien. Filosofía, Políticas, Estrategias y Experiencias Regionales Andinas.* Lima, Peru: Oxfam America.

Capel, H. (2016). Las ciencias sociales y el estudio del territorio. Biblio3W. *Revista Bilbiográfica de Geografía y Ciencias Sociales, XXI*(1.149). www.ub.edu/geocrit/b3w-1149.pdf

Castro-Gómez, S. (2000). Ciencias sociales, violencia epistémica y el problema de la invención del otro. In *La Colonialidad del Saber: Eurocentrismo y Ciencias Sociales: Perspectivas Latinoamericanas.* Buenos Aires: CLACSO, Consejo Latinoamericano de Ciencias Sociales. https://biblioteca.clacso.edu.ar/clacso/sur-sur/20100708045330/8_castro.pdf

CIDI. (2021). *Las Ciencias Sociales en Épocas de Crisis: Escenarios, Perspectivas y Exigencias en Tiempos de Pandemia.* Medellín, Colombia: Editorial Universidad Pontificia Bolivariana.

Contreras, G. (1995, Spring). Reseña de: "Hacia el origen del mito de la modernidad" de Enrique Dussel. *Política y Cultura*, no. 4, pp.217–221. redalyc.org/pdf/267/26700416.pdf

Copete, Y. A., Lozano, Á. E., & Valencia, C. K. (2020). La potencia y el lenguaje: Releer el Pacífico Colombiano. *Estudios del Pacífico, 1*(1), 11–37.

Da Silva Araújo, L., Da Silva Oliveira, I. B., & Rolack, J. S. (2014). Espiritualidad en la práctica de la terapia ocupacional: Interfaces en el campo de la ocupación humana. *Revista Electrónica Terapia Ocupacional Galicia, 11*(20). www.revistatog.com/num20/pdfs/revision3.pdf

Dussel, E. (2009, August 25). Una nueva edad en la historia de la filosofía: El diálogo mundial entre tradiciones filosóficas. *Tabula Rasa*, no. 11, pp.97–114. Bogotá, Colombia.

Dussel, E. (2020). *El Primer Debate Filosófico de la Modernidad* (1st edn). Buenos Aires: CLACSO Consejo Latinoamericano de Ciencias Sociales. https://biblioteca-repositorio.clacso.edu.ar/bitstream/CLACSO/15658/1/El-primer-debate.pdf

Dussel, E. D. (1994). *El Encubrimiento del Indio, 1492: Hacia el Origen del Mito de la Modernidad.* Mexico: Editorial Cambio XXI.

Echeverría, B. (2009). *¿Qué Es la Modernidad?* (1st edn). Mexico: Universidad Nacional Autónoma de México. https://libroschorcha.files.wordpress.com/2018/02/que-es-la-modernidad-bolivar-echeverria.pdf

Egan, M. (1997). The implicit spirituality of occupational therapy practice. *Canadian Journal of Occupational Therapy, 64*(3). https://doi.org/10.1177/000841749706400307

Escobar, A. (Ed.) (2014). *La Invención del Desarrollo* (2nd edn). Popayán, Colombia: Editorial Universidad del Cauca.

Escobar, A. (2016). Desde abajo, por la izquierda, y con la Tierra: La diferencia de Abya Yala/Afro/Latino/América. In *Pedagogías Decoloniales: Prácticas Insurgentes de Resistir*. 55.

Fals Borda, O. (2014). Prólogo a la primera edición. In A. Escobar (Ed.), *La Invención del Desarrollo* (D. Ochoa, Trans.), (2nd edn, pp. 43–45). Popayán, Colombia: Editorial Universidad del Cauca.

Gallegos Anda, C. E. (2018). Good living as a living law. *Australian Journal of Indigenous Education, 47*(1), 30–40.

Gómez Lillo, S., & Imperatore Blanche, E. (2021). Desarrollo de la terapia ocupacional en Latinoamérica. *Revista Chilena de Terapia Ocupacional, 22*(2), 207–217. https://doi.org/10.5354/0719-5346.2010.10566

Guajardo, A. (2016). Construcción de identidades, epistemes y prácticas en terapia ocupacional en América Latina. In S. Simó, A. Guajardo, O. F. Correa, S. M. Galheigo, & S. García (Eds.), *Terapias Ocupacionales desde el Sur: Derechos Humanos, Ciudadanía y Participación*. Universidad Santiago de Chile.

Gudynas, E., & Acosta, A. (2011). La renovación de la crítica al desarrollo y el Buen Vivir como alternativa. *Utopía y Praxis Latinoamericana, 16*(53), 71–83. www.redalyc.org/pdf/279/27919220007.pdf

Iwama, M. K., & Simó, S. (2008). El Modelo Kawa (Río). *TOG (A Coruña), 5*(2). www.revistatog.com/num8/pdfs/modelo2.pdf

Kuhn, T. (1971). *La Estructura de las Revoluciones Científicas*. Mexico: Fondo de Cultura. Económica.

Lozano, Á. E., & Copete, Y. A. (2019). La filosofía de vivir sabroso. *Revista Universidad de Antioquia*, 50–53.

Marques, T., & Roldan, M. (2020). Una reflexión crítica acerca del paradigma del "Buen Vivir" como alternativa al modelo de desarrollo. *Revista de Filosofía de la Universidad de Costa Rica, 59*(154), 59–67.

Martín-Baró, I. (1972). Del alcohol a la marihuana. *Colección Digital Ignacio Martín-Baró, 27*(283), 226–242. www.uca.edu.sv/coleccion-digital-IMB/articulo/del-alcohol-a-la-marihuana

MNICR. (2017, July). *Resumen de los Aportes Indígenas a la Política y Estrategia Nacional de Biodiversidad*. Mesa Nacional Indígena de Costa Rica. Costa Rica: Gobierno de Costa Rica.

Moruno, M. P., & Talavera, V. M. (2007). *Terapia Ocupacional: Una Perspectiva Histórica: 90 Años después de su Creación*. La Coruña: Revista TOG. www.revistatog.com/mono/num1/mono1_esp.pdf

Moya, R. (2009). La interculturalidad para todos en América Latina. In L. E. Lopéz (Ed.), *Interculturalidad, Educación y Ciudadanía: Perspectivas Latinoamericanas* (pp. 21–56). Plural Editores.

Navarrete, S. R. (2019). El tonto y los canallas. Notas para un republicanismo transmoderno. *Revista Stultifera, 2*(2), 135–139.

Pino, J. A., & Ulloa, F. (2016). Perspectiva crítica desde Latinoamérica: Hacia una desobediencia epistémica en terapia ocupacional contemporánea. *Cadernos de Terapia Ocupacional da UFSCar, 24*(2), 421–427.

Porto-Gonçalves, C. W., & Rego-Monteiro, C. L. (2022). De la geopolítica y la política en tiempos de caos sistémico: Una mirada desde América Latina/Abya Yala. *Revista Especializada En Estudios Latinoamericanos, 8*(16), 192–216. https://dialnet.unirioja.es/servlet/articulo?codigo=8475358

Ramírez, O. D., Satizabal, R. M., Rojas, C. C., & García, R. S. (2022). Comprensiones de lo comunitario en Terapia Ocupacional: Aproximaciones desde la Revista Ocupación Humana, 1996–2021. *Revista Ocupación Humana, 22*(Suppl.), 102–116. https://doi.org/10.25214/25907816.1342

Rivera Cusicanqui, S. (2011). Entre el Buen Vivir y el desarrollo: Una perspectiva indianista. In I. Errejón & A. Serrano (Eds.), *¡Ahora Es Cuándo, Carajo! Del Asalto a la Transformación del Estado en Bolivia* (pp. 169–180). España: Ediciones de Intervención Popular. El Viejo Topo.

Robles, F. (2012, December). Epistemologías de la modernidad: Entre el etnocentrismo, el racionalismo universalista y las alternativas latinoamericanas. *Cinta de Moebio*, no. 45, 169–203. www.redalyc.org/articulo.oa?id=10125104001

Rodríguez, S. A. (2016). *Teoría y práctica del Buen Vivir: Orígenes, debates conceptuales, y conflictos sociales. El caso de Ecuador.* Doctoral thesis, University of the Basque Country. https://filosofiadelbuenvivir.com/wp-content/uploads/2016/09/Tesis-Doctoral-Buen-Vivir-Adriana-Rodr%C3%ADguez-S.pdf

Rojas, C. P. (2011). *Ocupación: Sentido, Realización y Libertad. Diálogos Ocupacionales en Torno al Sujeto, la Sociedad y el Medio Ambiente.* Bogotá: Universidad Nacional de Colombia. https://repositorio.unal.edu.co/bitstream/handle/unal/9033/9789587197297.pdf?se

Sajed, A. (2020, July 27). From the Third World to the Global South. E-International Relations. www.e-ir.info/2020/07/27/from-the-third-world-to-the-global-south

Santacruz, M. L. (2002). La dimensión espiritual en terapia ocupacional. *Revista de la Ocupación Humana, 9*(4), 52–60. https://latinjournal.org/index.php/roh/article/download/652/567/1554

Sarango, F. (2010). La interculturalidad como práctica de vida y la educación superior como diálogo de saberes. Las políticas Públicas Interculturales desde la Visión de los Pueblos Indígenas. Vídeo Foro. San José, Costa Rica.

Tribunal Constitucional del Ecuador. Asamblea Constituyente. (2008). *Nueva Constitución Política del Ecuador.*

UNESCO. (2022). *Ancestral System of Knowledge of the Four Indigenous Peoples, Arhuaco, Kankuamo, Kogui and Wiwa of the Sierra Nevada de Santa Marta.* UNESCO Intangible Cultural Heritage. https://ich.unesco.org/en/RL/ancestral-system-of-knowledge-of-the-four-indigenous-peoples-arhuaco-kankuamo-kogui-and-wiwa-of-the-sierra-nevada-de-santa-marta-01886

Vélez, M. (2022, July 13). Entrevista [Interview]. Interviewed by F. Rocha, Colombia (personal communication).

Vindas-Acosta, J., & Valdelomar-Marín, E. (2021). Cambio de perspectiva en los paradigmas y prácticas profesionales en el acompañamiento de personas que usan sustancias psicoactivas: Análisis desde la psicología y la terapia ocupacional. *Revista Terapéutica, 15*(1), 119–133.

Waldmüller, J. M. (2014). Buen vivir, Sumak kawsay, "Good living": An introduction and overview. *Alternautas, 1*(1), 17–25.

WFOT. (2010). *Position Statement on Diversity and Culture.* World Federation of Occupational Therapy.

PART 2

IDENTITIES

CHAPTER 3

The Ethnic-Racial Issue in Occupational Therapy Training

CONTRIBUTIONS FROM ABYA YALA

Cristian Valderrama Nuñez, Lina Carla Chambilla Tarqui, Jaqueline Cruz Perdomo, and Magno Nunes Farias

Abstract

This chapter aims to critically reflect and systematize some anti-racist practices in occupational therapy found in Abya Yala, the name of our land, which colonialists called Latin America. This chapter is based on the need to incorporate the ethnic-racial category, given its relevance to the configuration of human occupations and everyday activities. Additionally, it aims to identify the anti-racist practices that this profession needs to embrace in our territories. To date, we analyzed the occupational therapy literature to identify the presence and/or absence of ethnic-racial discourses in our field. We particularly focused on the professional training of occupational therapists in South America. It is also proposed that within the knowledge held by Black and Indigenous peoples, there exist forms of knowledge that enlighten the profession, as they are forms of resistance to the capitalist-colonial-patriarchal-racist matrix in which occupational therapy is situated. To create this chapter, we conducted a narrative review of articles published in online journals specialized in occupational therapy in South America. The analysis was carried out by searching for relevant keywords. We included some formative experiences of the authors of this text in their respective spaces of professional development.

Keywords

occupational therapy; professional training; racism; ethnic-racial; race

Learning outcomes

- Critically analyze and synthesize the current research on ethnic-racial issues and racism published in South American occupational therapy journals, identifying key themes, gaps, and areas for future study.
- Examine how racism and ethnic discrimination manifest in occupational therapy education and practice, highlighting the urgent need for deeper engagement with these issues across the profession.
- Describe specific educational experiences, curricula, and practices that meaningfully incorporate ethnic-racial content and anti-racist approaches in occupational therapy programs.
- Explore how systemic racism impacts occupational therapy and propose strategies for creating more inclusive and equitable educational and practice environments.

Introduction

Our profession has developed from a colonial perspective, where the naturalization of Eurocentric and English-speaking knowledge and practices has led us to perceive them as our own, disregarding the contextual conditions that determine local communities' existence, presence, and behavior. This results in the inability to recognize the knowledge and ways of understanding the world specific to our region.

Additionally, this implies that occupational therapy disregards the history of colonization and the different mechanisms of oppression experienced by subordinate social groups. In this regard, Beagan et al. (2022b) denounce systemic and epistemic racism within occupational therapy, as evaluations, theories, models, and frameworks being taught and practiced in occupational therapy that only consider the White-mixed and Western/North-Western understanding of the world. Problematizing the ethnic-racial issue during professional training is of utmost urgency. Doing so can raise awareness about knowledge that can challenge racism and promote anti-racist practices in occupational therapy.

According to Hopenhayn and Bello (2001), discussing the ethnic-racial issue reveals the historical discrimination process experienced by a significant part of our population. This exclusion is based on race and ethnicity. One is based on skin color; the other is related to the cultural aspects of native peoples. Consequently, due to our population characteristics, both notions are indivisible and intersectional with other forms of exclusion in the capitalist-patriarch-colonial system. The root of this situation is the alleged supremacy one particular social group (colonists) has over other groups (colonized) that hinders and excludes access to certain rights and to reaping the benefits of a supportive and united economy with Mother Earth. It hinders the joyous living of Native and Black peoples.

Understanding this issue is crucial, since this condition hinders participation in occupations and daily activities important to the individuals and communities racialized by cultural, social, and institutional exclusion mechanisms imposed by dominant groups. Disclosing the ethnic-racial category is a political and ethical vindication for the African-descent and ethnic communities forming our territory. This action aims to do everything we can to dignify their occupations.

In colonial times, Europe named our territory "Spanish America." By the mid-19th century, it was renamed "Latin America" by the White-mixed elite (Ayala Mora, 2013). Many authors have challenged this invasion of how we recognize ourselves as a community. One of them is Lélia Gonzáles, who, from a Black-Indigenous feminist perspective, renamed our territory "Améfrica Ladina" during the 1970s (Gomez Correal, 2020). Since the 1990s, the Indigenous and Black movements have also rejected the European denomination of our territories, condemning the Spanish and Portuguese invasion. This leads to the vindication of Abya Yala, the name of our territory taken from the Gunadule or Kuna people living in Colombia and Panamá. These two denominations frequently appear in decolonial literature and popular movements. For instance, we find references to this topic in Ruth Lozano Lerma (2019) and Mara Viveros Vigoya (2021).

The starting point for the discussion of the ethnic-racial issue in occupational therapy

To identify the presence or absence of ethnic-racial discourses within our profession, we reviewed academic production in online journals specialized in occupational therapy in our region based on a narrative review characterized by more open search criteria. This step is essential since these studies have valuable information that can be transmitted to students through diverse teaching methods during their training programs.

We reviewed the following journals: the *Chilean Journal of Occupational Therapy* (*RECHTO*, acronym in Spanish); *ContexTO*; the *Occupational Therapy Student's Journal* (*RETO*, acronym in Spanish); the *Brazilian Interinstitutional Journal of Occupational Therapy* (*REVISBRATO*, acronym in Portuguese); the *Occupational Therapy Journal* of São Paulo University; *Cadernos Brasileiros of Occupational Therapy*; the *Argentinian Journal of Occupational Therapy*; and *Human Occupation Journal* (*Revista Ocupación Humana* in Spanish; Colombia).

We want to clarify that, for this chapter, we purposefully decided not to include texts from other databases such as Web of Science, Scopus, SciELO, or other occupational therapy journals with authorship from continents outside our region, where the topic of discussion is Abya Yala. We did not include conference proceedings or institutional repositories containing papers from undergraduate and postgraduate students.

The keywords we used in our search were: racism, race, racialization, ethnicity, native peoples, Black population, migration, and Indigenous. This decision was based on yielding as many results as possible to identify academic production involving the ethnic-racial category, characterized by a narrative review. We obtained 28 articles distributed, as shown in Table 3.1.

Table 3.1 Number of articles published in Abya Yala journals about the ethnic-racial category

Country	Journal	URL	Number of articles
Chile	Occupational Therapy Student's Journal	https://reto.ubo.cl/index.php/reto	1
	ContexTO	www.revistacontextoucen.cl/index.php/contexto/about	1
	Chilean Journal of Occupational Therapy	https://revistaterapiaocupacional.uchile.cl	2
Brazil	Brazilian Interinstitutional Journal of Occupational Therapy	https://revistas.ufrj.br/index.php/ribto	7
	Cadernos Brasileiros of Occupational Therapy Journal	https://www.scielo.br/j/cadbto/	13
	Occupational Therapy Journal of São Paulo University	www.revistas.usp.br/rto/index	1
Colombia	Human Occupation Journal	https://latinjournal.org/index.php/roh/index	3
Argentina	Argentinian Journal of Occupational Therapy	https://revista.terapia-ocupacional.org.ar	0
Total			28

Among the articles reviewed, 19 of them met the criteria to be included in this study. The remaining nine documents included the criteria but centered their content around other topics. Most academic research concerning the ethnic-racial category in the consulted journals dates from 2022 onwards.

This indicates that the disciplinary interest in this topic is recent. Most of the articles included in our review are from Brazilian journals, comprising 78.9% (n = 15). This was followed by three articles published in Chilean journals (15.8%) and one published in the Colombian journal (5.3%). As shown in Table 3.1, one journal had no articles related to the topic. Regarding the year of publication, the articles are distributed in the following way: 73.7% (n = 14) were published between 2020 and 2021, 21.0% (n = 4) were published between 2016 and 2018, and only one (5.3%) publication in 2022.

The following provides a synthesis of the main topics of the analyzed texts. This is displayed according to the country in which the paper was published, as our objective is to highlight academic research from specialized Abya Yala publications in the Chilean, Brazilian, and Colombian journals focused on an ethnic-racial category.

Chilean publications

A lack of academic production in occupational therapy concerning the State–Mapuche issue and the necessity of a platform to reflect on racial issues in occupational therapy training

The analysis of Chilean journals reveals a lack of attention to the historical conflict between the Chilean State and the Mapuche[1] people. This conflict encompasses a history of abuse, rights violations, and the pursuit of self-determination for the Mapuche nation. The analysis also evidences the experiences of other ethnic groups. At the same time, articles in Chile showcase suggestions made by Brazilian authors that mainly focus on racial aspects. Subsequently, we present three texts: the first two discuss the racial problem and its relevance in academic training; the third one addresses the issue of ethnicity and its effects on the childhood of Mapuche children.

Ambrosio et al. (2021) suggest that occupations can perpetuate systemic and institutional racism. As a response, they propose some ideas regarding anti-racist practices in occupational therapy. The representation of different colors in toys that resemble the human body and materials used for interventions with kids, the use of games, music, and some artistic rituals or ceremonies from the Indigenous and Black people's worldview might be helpful to decolonize the occupational therapists.

In the professional training field, the authors suggest that including the

1 The Mapuche people are one of the Indigenous peoples of Southern Chile. Their relationship with the Chilean state is characterized by the latter legitimizing the usurpation of their sacred lands, violating and destroying their worldview. In this context, the Mapuche people represent resistance and struggle to preserve their traditions and protect their territory, which has been expressed since the period of the Spanish conquest in Chile in the 16th century.

topic of racism as elemental content in the first years of studying is fundamental. This would enable us to train professionals who respect diversities and differences, allowing them to identify the richness of the Indigenous worldview and the African-descent knowledge.

Farias, Leite, and Amorim (2020) provide a historical review of how the ethnic-racial issue, particularly Blackness, has been addressed in occupational therapy in Latin America and other parts of the world, including its expression in professional training. The authors demonstrate that despite the progress made at incorporating social aspects into professional training, racial and ethnic relationships and issues related to Black people and racial equality have been overlooked. Not even the World Federation of Occupational Therapists (WFOT) has included these categories in the basic training of occupational therapists, nor have they included it in their research priorities. The authors also emphasize the necessity of developing anti-racist practices that include intersectional actions involving social groups outside of the Black community, and stress the importance of the articulating social role of occupational therapists.

Fuentes et al. (2020) investigated the effects of political violence in games played by Mapuche children in the Araucanía region. Their study shows that Mapuche children play for enjoyment and that, in this occupation, they reproduce the violent experiences they have been exposed to. The authors of this study encourage readers to connect with the topic of political violence from a social perspective in the field of occupational therapy, which allows addressing issues from a human-rights perspective. It is important to note that the sample of this study is children from Native groups, unlike the previous studies. However, this study does not extensively explore the ethnic-racial issue as a category that considers historically oppressed groups.

Brazilian publications

A focus on Blackness in health, higher education, and possible intervention practices

The first work identified in Brazilian periodicals is Barros (2002) about the itineraries of madness in Dogon territory (West African society). The author discusses her field research carried out between 1994 and 1996 in the Dogon lands, Black African society of the Republic of Mali (West Africa), stating that "it is observed that the Dogon society has a significant lexicon linked to the designation and understanding of madness" (Barros, 2002, p. 64). It is understood that the itineraries of madness in this society can be different, which can involve reception, social reintegration, or even imprisonment at home and abandonment.

Pastore and Sato (2018) present an overview of academic research in social occupational therapy that has interfaced with the theme of Africa. The authors emphasize that the productions are pioneered by the work since the beginning of the 2000s by Denise Dias Barros (Barros, 2002). The text announces and debates studies that discuss actions within the scope of research and practice, which bring themes about ways of life, migration, public policies, childhood, gender, mobility, racism, and xenophobia, among other topics involving African immigrants in Brazil. Based on the perspective of valuing African culture and themes, ethnography is an important tool for carrying out research connecting Africa and social occupational therapy, crossed by the issue of cultural diversity.

Perilla et al. (2021) researched the Kankuamo people in the Caribbean region of Colombia. Their study focused on the importance of COVID-19, its effects on intercultural healthcare, and how it is related to death, considering the virus mortality rate. The authors showcase the stories of three members of the Kankuamo community and establish connections between these narratives and the understanding of human occupation as an intermediary of the diverse social, spiritual, and ecological symbolical dimensions within the Indigenous worldview concerning the virus. Their study addresses methodological challenges for future research, emphasizing the need to avoid epistemic appropriation or misappropriation of knowledge to genuinely respect the participants' narratives. This work dialogues with the work of Macedo et al. (2016), which analyzes occupational therapy practices within the Guaraní Indigenous community of Espirito Santo (Brazil), bringing contributions to the profession's role in cultural contexts and the sphere of ethnicity. The analysis concerns the strengthening of human actions and the affirmation of identities that involve actions essential for producing knowledge and for theoretical-methodological and professional training in social occupational therapy and cultural contexts.

Leite, Farias, and Martins (2021) highlight the contributions of Ivone Lara, a Black woman who was a cultural producer, samba performer, nurse, social worker, and occupational therapy specialist (at that time, the year 1940, this profession did not exist in Brazil since other professionals undertook an equivalent role). She played a significant role in occupational therapy practices starting from the 1940s in Brazil, alongside Nise da Silveira,[2] in proposing humanized care for institutionalized individuals in asylums. Their practices included visiting the home and families of hospitalized individuals

2 Nise da Silveira worked alongside Ivone Lara in 1940 in Brazil, implementing revolutionary practices based on art and the humanization of care for institutionalized individuals with mental disorders. This occurred in a context where the dominant Brazilian psychiatry relied on reductionist scientific and technological methods, such as electroshock and neurological surgery (Castro & Lima, 2007).

and using music (samba) as a therapeutic treatment. Lara contributed to advancing humanized care in multi/inter/transdisciplinary approaches and community settings, recognizing the importance of integrating them with popular knowledge/cultures. For the authors, telling her story is a manifestation of recognition and retrieval of Black memories in the discipline, which have been denied, even distorted.

Valério et al. (2021) identify racist practices in universities and the difficulties they create for Black female students. They found that the main issue for the students was their sense of not belonging in university spaces. The students identified university spaces as hostile and segregating. Their experiences of prejudice and discrimination were mainly shown covertly, through disdainful glances or treatment, in university halls, locations for practical classes, and internship sites. Finally, these stories evidence Black women's difficult task of overcoming the servile image historically associated with their skin color, gender, social status, and sexuality. This stereotype often persists regardless of the spaces they occupy, their work, or their intellectual achievements.

The strategies for resistance that female Black students use against racism in university spaces include the emotional support lent by their friends, creating spaces on campus to feel represented, and fostering discussions about the experiences of Black individuals in politics and higher education. This serves to fight against prejudice and racial discrimination. Through these efforts, moments can be created that allow Black students to reclaim their identity with pride.

Regarding the experiences of African university students in Brazil, Bezerra and Alves (2022) suggest that higher education institutions need to create better welcoming mechanisms for Black immigrant students. By doing so, these students can have more satisfactory experiences, enhance their sense of belonging, and increase their social participation. The absence of such experiences can harm their adaptation process and affect other areas, such as health and academic performance. Occupational therapists can incorporate these aspects as guiding elements in interventions and when creating spaces for experience, knowledge, and culture exchange. By doing so, they can encourage transformations in university spaces, fostering inclusion, plurality, and authentic diversity.

Ambrosio and Silva (2022) discuss the concept of intersectionality and its contribution to analyzing different forms of oppression directed toward Black bodies and other heteronormative expressions imposed by hegemonic colonial patriarchal and capitalist forces, such as racism, among others. The authors encourage us to consider the domination matrix and processes within occupational therapy attention groups to understand better the complexity of everyday life and occupations that have been conditioned by historical sociocultural and political colonialism. The concept of intersectionality would enrich the practical knowledge in occupational therapy as it considers identity components, relationships, and interactions.

França, Queiroz, and Bezerra (2016) discuss research conducted in the *terreiro de candomblé*[3] *Casa de Iemanjá IyáOgun-Té* and in a Family Healthcare Unit, both located in the same working-class neighborhood, which has been predominantly Black, in the local government of Maceió (Alagoas, Brazil). The purpose of the study was to contribute to the establishment of the occupational therapist's role in mediating the necessary dialogues for the implementation of the National Comprehensive Health Policy for the Black Population[4] (PNSIPN, in Portuguese). The study yielded two categories: (a) the relationship between the people adhering to *candomblé* and the topics and spaces for healthcare; and (b) the perspective of health professionals about users and the PNSIPN, both focused on the people from *terreiro*. The results showed that *candomblé* adherents found it easier to navigate various health spaces, choosing the *terreiro* as a place of reception and resolution for processes aimed at promoting health balance. On the part of healthcare professionals, there was a lack of awareness about the sociocultural context of the users and the affirmative policies of the Brazilian Unified Health System for the *terreiro* people.

Farias, Leite, and Costa (2018) reflect on the subordination processes that taint Black people's existence and hinder the affirmation of the Black identity, which is directly connected to occupational apartheid's exclusionary structures. The authors offer a historical and contemporary view of the Black population in Brazil, enabling us to consider the possibilities of occupational therapy with these individuals. The occupational therapist is recognized as a political and social agent who can help with emancipation activities, in groups or individually, to pursue awareness and empower these individuals. Interventions should be grounded in valuing Afro-Brazilian identities.

Amorim et al. (2020) wrote "Social asphyxias" about the hardships of the Black population and the role of occupational therapy. Their study aimed to provoke a reaction in occupational therapists by introducing the

---

3 A place where rituals of *candomblé* are performed, a religion of the African diaspora that developed in Brazil, as well as other Afro-Brazilian religions.

4 The National Comprehensive Health Policy for the Black Population is a public policy articulated by the Ministry of Health of Brazil, approved in 2006. It contains principles, guidelines, and strategies aimed at improving the health conditions of the Brazilian Black population, which the Unified Health System must implement.

concept of "everyday racism" and how it affects their practices and academic production regarding Black people. The authors approach the reality of Black people as being marked by the concepts of social asphyxia and children and young people's genocide, triggering social movements like Black Lives Matter worldwide, including in Brazil. In this way, it becomes evident that the context of racism, tied to the depths of inequality and triggered by the COVID-19 pandemic, leads to a death policy targeted at the Black population, which unfortunately had a boom during the Bolsonaro regime.

The authors highlight the increasing number of professionals turning to this topic, enabling the construction of diverse knowledge about and for the Black population and the technical-political actions for occupational therapy. Finally, they point out that the anti-racist practice of occupational therapy is an ethical, political, and technical determinant for carrying out actions that envision racial and social justice in the lives of Black and non-Black individuals in a racialized society.

Costa et al. (2020) gathered data representing the African Studies Lab and the Lab-Ịṣẹ́ occupational therapy activities at the Federal University of Rio de Janeiro, Brazil. Lab-Ịṣẹ́ is dedicated to activities from African and Afro-Brazilian perspectives to mend the historical debt that violated their rights and dismiss the singularities of these groups. The authors provide an overview of the ethnic-racial issue in occupational therapy programs in Brazil. They conclude that the data signals the importance of questioning how the spaces in occupational therapy training are perceived about racism (against or reproducing it). They point out that by not including mandatory courses that delve into ethnic-racial issues, occupational therapy programs may be perpetuating racism within the profession (Costa et al., 2020, p. 739).

Fernandes et al. (2021) further contribute to this discussion by presenting a case study of occupational therapy practice in the Institutional Service for the Reception of Children and Adolescents in São Paulo. Their study analyzed the experiences of children and adolescents in institutionalization processes. A counter-hegemonic proposal for action emerges from a decolonial and critical occupational therapy perspective. This proposal values and acknowledges Black cultural identity within the field as a form of practice that is Afro-referent and anti-racist, promoting positive change in occupational therapy.

> [I]n daily living activities, the occupational therapy professional seeks to view human activities from a Black perspective, as well as to show appreciation for

> the environment of Black communities and their family life, where racism exists, as well as in the *quilombo*.[5] (Fernandes et al., 2021, p. 637)

Cruz, Barradas, and Sampaio (2021) conducted a qualitative-descriptive study in the peripheral community of Belém (in Pará, Brazil), where children volunteered and participated in the "Afrocine Social Project." The exercise aimed to broaden their leisure space and cultural enrichment by screening films, audiovisual content, and games. This study aimed to understand the significance of engaging in the Afrocine Project for Black children and volunteers from the peripheral community of Belém and its impact on their lives. The study reveals the importance of education, representation, and Black consciousness in this environment, distraught by the injustice caused by racism. The study results revealed that children perceive the activities in the project as essential for their lives and personal development. They consider these activities, such as education and play, fundamental. However, the study concludes that there is a lack of content regarding practices and training directed toward Black people, particularly children.

Farias and Vicente (2022) describe and analyze a practice that occupational therapists and psychologists use. Their study focused on a group activity where young Black and non-Black university students participated. The name of the activity was "Black bodies in university: Dialogs to confront institutional racism." It is stated that the activity created a moment of dialogue and reflection, fostering latent issues in our social and racial dynamics and seeking to strengthen anti-racist practices through empowerment and awareness movements. In their interdisciplinary action, it concludes that occupational therapy and psychology can foster spaces in universities for critical debate on social issues.

Colombian publications

A focus on Indigenous problems and a neglect of the occupational knowledge of Black people

Rojas (2017) encourages Colombian occupational therapists to consider in their practice that Colombia is a multi-ethnic country and that it is necessary to share the experiences of those affected by violent practices from a decolonial perspective. The presence of armed and social conflict has been incessant in the country's history, disrupting the lives of rural, Indigenous,

---

5 *Quilombos* are territories conquered by a group of enslaved Africans who fought for their freedom, resisting forced labor and dehumanization. Historically, they are characterized as spaces of struggle, resistance, and appreciation of African and Afro-Brazilian culture.

and Afro-Colombian communities. This leads to forms of disability and changes in the customary occupations of its inhabitants, it disrupts spirituality and constantly displaces the population from their territory. This is why occupational therapists must focus on rural communities, the underprivileged communities, by working in territories from the *sentipensar*[6] of these communities. Although the text is related to the topic, this study does not go in-depth about the ethnic-racial category in occupational therapy.

Points of reflection on the ethnic-racial issue in Abya Yala

As a result of the narrative review, two main questions emerge to deepen the analysis regarding the ethnic-racial category in occupational therapy, which are briefly answered below.

What challenges are posed to include the ethnic-racial category in disciplinary education?

There is a lack of specific training experiences in occupational therapy that address the ethnic-racial issue. The same applies to the available learning methods and their potential effects when training professionals. Although the epistemologies of Black and Indigenous peoples in our countries are particularly rich in occupations for the care of life (that is, in human activities that protect the balance between human beings, as well as between them and nature, to sustain and respect the life of all living beings on the planet, such as food sovereignty, Indigenous education, midwifery, and artisanal mining, among others), this knowledge of occupational life is not part of occupational therapy education. Universities must recognize, from a critical intercultural perspective, the significance of racial diversity and the necessity to integrate Black and Indigenous knowledge to promote a pluralistic society. By doing so, universities can evolve into safe and inclusive spaces, fulfilling their social responsibility. However, achieving this requires interdisciplinary efforts to be made. This should aim at a broader integration of cultural and epistemological perspectives, a question that requires students, authorities, and teachers to highlight the importance of a genuine dialogue between the different actors involved,

---

6 *Sentipensar* is a notion of Indigenous and rural origin used in the community of Chiapas, Mexico. It refers to the integrated way of thinking and feeling in our everyday practices, where thoughts and emotions are not separated into two distinct worlds. The rural community in the Colombian Caribbean also uses it to describe how thoughts and feelings are interconnected in daily life, forming a unity. *Sentipensar* represents a departure from the dichotomous thinking often encountered in the Western knowledge approach.

so that the situations that produce violations, such as social class, rurality, machismo, and xenophobia, among others, can be critically addressed and mitigated through concrete institutional actions. It is important that university institutions get involved to promote the creation of truly innovative and inclusive strategies that become shared resources for all and produce rich diversity.

Why is it essential to document anti-racist practices in occupational therapy?

Because documented anti-racist practices are missing as a crucial issue, we need occupational therapy studies focused on Native peoples or First Nations, particularly occupational therapy interventions in those groups.

There have been no shared studies under Black or Indigenous people's authorship related to occupational therapy. We have a long way to go in the dialogue of knowledge and concrete actions that allow the recognition of other ways of being, existing, and doing. Regarding professional training, including ethnic-racial issues as essential content in the first years is fundamental. Not doing so could cause or reproduce racist practices in the field, perpetuating the subordination of these social groups.

Documenting anti-racist practices in occupational therapy is crucial since it enables us to identify this profession's contributions to the well-being of historically compromised communities. At the same time, this exercise becomes an opportunity to incorporate new disciplinary knowledge and practices that are more socially fitting and can decolonize the disciplinary bases as an opening political act to new horizons. It is essential to say that to progress toward decolonized occupational therapy, we must consider that the discipline operates in a colonized world. Thus, there is a constant risk of the discipline being compromised by its most powerful environment, emphasizing the need for continuous reflective action.

Experiences concerning the professional training of occupational therapists in the ethnic-racial topic

It is important to consider that Abya Yala is under a constant migratory process that can cause personal and cultural changes in individuals with whom occupational therapy cooperates and interacts so that they obtain the expected benefits of their participation. This is a situation that future occupational therapists should be aware of. At the same time, incorporating the ethnic-racial issue in occupational therapy training would enable the development of professionals with greater awareness and critical capacity when facing situations of vulnerability and social exclusion, as experienced by racialized individuals in our territories. It is also an opportunity to progress in the decolonization of education, thereby constructing intervention alternatives relevant to our region's social and material reality while respecting and dignifying the identities of our people.

Below, we include our personal experiences concerning the ethnic-racial category in the formative processes in which we are immersed. Our objective is to complement the narrative review we previously presented and provide experiences that can inspire its inclusion in those formative programs that have not yet considered it.

The occupational therapy program at the Universidad Mayor de San Andrés in Bolivia

In 2010, the Universidad Mayor of San Andrés (hereinafter UMSA) started the first-ever professional training program for occupational therapists in the Plurinational State of Bolivia through its Faculty of Medicine in La Paz. It is important to mention that this is the only higher education institution training occupational therapists in this country.

This project was promoted thanks to the collaboration of the Japanese and Chilean governments. Both countries support the Bolivian Healthcare Ministry in training rehabilitation professionals with an inclusive perspective. This alliance emerges from the need to equalize opportunities and balance access to public health services in the country.

By the end of March 2010, we had only 20 students in our first year of the program. Due to this, university authorities decided that occupational therapy and speech therapy students should share subjects and spaces during their first years of training. The curriculum would include common subjects that later became unique and innovative compared to the rest of the university system in the country. To add more human resources to the rehabilitation field, both majors train professionals capable of the sanitary demand in rehabilitation for a population of more than 95,884 people with some type of disability (Defensoría del Pueblo, 2019). Bolivia is a diverse, multi-ethnic, and multiracial country in reclaiming human rights and recognizing and respecting its cultural values.

Concerning the conceptual competencies in professional occupational therapy training in Bolivia (Universidad Mayor de San Andrés, 2019), the program encourages the construction of new knowledge to interpret biological, social, cultural, environmental, and psychological factors that affect individuals, families, and communities. The discussion of individual, local, regional, and national needs in healthcare to benefit communities considers cultural, political, social, and economic differences, as well as the abilities of people with and without disabilities.

Regarding technical competencies, the occupational therapist implements actions to care for individuals, families, and groups. However, human competencies stand out during training since they encourage the development of integral activities that facilitate communication, interaction, and intervention productively by considering the sociocultural characteristics of each region and population of the country.

One distinctive feature that can be found in the Bolivian occupational therapy program is the implementation of courses that prepare the student in sanitary practices and knowledge that values ethnic knowledge for the adequate service of the diverse Bolivian population. During their first year of school, students take a class in Native Language, in which they learn about grammar and how to communicate with people from the native Aimara community.

There is also a subject called "Traditional Bolivian Medicine" for developing fundamental knowledge about reassessing ancestral knowledge and practices from the perspectives and values of different nations and rural Indigenous peoples. The program also teaches sign language, another class where students develop communication skills with people with hearing impairment.

The occupational therapy program at the Andrés Bello University in Concepción, Chile

The occupational therapy program at the Andrés Bello University, a private institution, is imparted simultaneously in Chile's three biggest cities, referred to as institutional branches: Viña del Mar, Santiago, and Concepción. This program aims to educate professionals of excellence, deeply committed to social issues, enthusiastic, and equipped with critical-thinking skills from a perspective of values and ethics based on human rights and respect for diversity. The program aims to promote the well-being of individuals and communities through occupations directed to compromised groups, people with disabilities, or with difficulties related to their occupations. This way, professionals will contribute to a more participatory, inclusive, and fair society (Universidad Andrés Bello, 2017).

Considering what has just been said, and due to the concern of some professors from the program in the Concepción branch, some content about the ethnic-racial category has been included preliminarily in some courses in the study program.

This motivation arises from the need to update the discussion of the ethnic-racial issue in professional training, considering the national context of the constituent process and its discussion in the occupational therapy and occupational sciences field. In addition, Chile has turned into a critical migration pole in the southern cone in the last few years. This implies a responsibility to understand migration and its impact on daily life, healthcare, education, and social protection.

The Community Health class is taught in the first year of the program, encompassing four teaching hours divided into instructive and workshop hours. The class concerns the concept of intercultural health, focusing on native peoples' worldview about health and well-being and interculturality's contribution to strengthening support for immigrants in the healthcare field (Altmann, 2016; Pérez, Nazar, & Cova, 2016). In the same year, in a class called Society, Culture, and Occupation, students can recognize different social and cultural settings and how the construction of human subjectivity and the understanding of occupation converge from a historical, social, and cultural point of view. To achieve this, in other program classes, students learn about ethnicity and Native peoples, considering the similarities and differences between multiculturalism and interculturality.

During the second year of the program, after finishing the class Theoretical Perspectives II, students are expected to be able to discuss and recognize the different theoretical approaches that represent occupational therapies, with emphasis on those that contribute with social, critical, ethical, and political perspectives. One class, An Antiracist Occupational Therapy, teaches students about systemic racism and how it is found in the discipline. They also learn about the strategies that have been developed to overcome racism and how occupational therapists must include this category in their knowledge to be able to create anti-racist practices (Beagan et al., 2022a, 2002b; Leite et al., 2021). Finally, in the program's third year, students take a class named Mental Health I. Its main topic is the concept of intersectionality, and the interaction between mental health problems and the racialization process of the Latin American migration in Chile is studied in depth with particular attention to the relation between acculturation processes and the negative psychosocial impact of racial marginalization and exclusion.

It is important to note that despite these experiences, evaluating the meaning and significance students attribute to these topics in their professional training is still necessary.

A Colombian experience—accompaniment program for pedagogical processes from a diverse approach

Next, we present an interdisciplinary experience[7] involving speech therapy, occupational therapy, and popular education[8] in the Indigenous community of the Honduras ward in the local government of Morales, Cauca Department, Colombia, in 2014.

The initiative was inspired by the interests of the schools to obtain information about the development conditions of Indigenous students with disabilities and, in general, of all the students to strengthen their teaching practices. In addition, this sparked the interest of professionals from the University of Valle and the El Patio Collective to learn about the knowledge and education of the Nasa people in the Mesón community and to understand other teaching practices and their possible dialogues with occupational therapy, speech therapy, and popular education fields.

This experience was called "accompaniment program for pedagogical processes from a diverse approach." It was divided into four parts: screening of students from preschool to fifth grade of primary school in Mixed Rural Honduras School, Lomitas School, San José School, and El Mesón and Chorrera Blanca School; accompaniment for teachers; discussion group with families; and finally, inhabiting the territory. The main events are described further in Table 3.2.

Some of the lessons learned from these experiences are:

- Professionals in the field of disability must challenge the established truths in their professions and shift toward the *sentipensar* from the community's territories. We need to question our professional training, primarily since we work with individuals labeled as "people with disabilities" by the discourse of modernity. Additionally, we must consider their role in indigenous self-education and their community.

- To work with and within the community, we must walk through the territory, avoiding judgment of values. This entails listening and engaging in dialogue with everyone in the community, being open to

7 From the El Patio Collective and the University of Valle, we were involved in designing and implementing the entire proposal at the Indigenous Educational Institution El Mesón. The speech therapists were Jefferson López and Mauricio Varela, the popular educator Francisco Javier Medina, and the occupational therapists Karen Caicedo and Jaqueline Cruz.

8 Popular education is a type of education that combines awareness of the sociopolitical conditions in which people carry out their daily lives, with the intention that they themselves can transform them in search of their emancipation and individual and collective well-being.

being questioned by communal Indigenous knowledge and practices, sharing the community's everyday life and special events, and getting involved in their spirituality to work with children and their teachers.

- Documenting our experience, socializing with the community, and maintaining photographic records of their daily lives proved valuable. Additionally, creating therapy documentation notes, planning, and the intervention results were beneficial. Writing and reading *coplas* (traditional poetic verses), songs, listening to the children's stories in the school, and consulting Indigenous bibliographic material played a significant role in documenting our experiences.

In the context of occupational therapy, it is essential to recognize that our work in Indigenous communities goes beyond the prevailing theories and models of our profession in education. This knowledge cannot be solely obtained from institutional settings at universities. To truly transform our professional practice, being receptive and open to learning from the Indigenous community is crucial. This entails establishing a horizontal dialogue with the knowledge held by the children and teachers within the Indigenous education system.

Table 3.2 The journey of the "accompaniment program for pedagogical processes from a diverse approach" experience

Integral development screening	Traditional games: Grandma's Chest for preschool and first grade and The Round of the Wolf for second through fifth grade. Task analysis with the analysis matrix of mathematical, social, language, movement, and scientific knowledge. Description of the games: • Grandma's Chest is a circle game in which one player gives a "jewel" to the others by pretending to give it away. However, they only pass it to one player. In the end, another player guesses who has the "jewel," realizing it through the gestures or attitudes of their companions, considering that they can be deceitful or evident. • The Round of the Wolf is a circle game in which a refrain is sung with questions and answers between the wolf and a group of children; when they finish singing, the wolf goes out to chase the children until it reaches one, and then the game ends.

Writing development screening	Narrative text: The stories "Niña Bonita" (Pretty Girl) for second and third grade, "El Tigre y el Ratón" (The Tiger and the Mouse) for fourth and fifth. Analysis of written language and comprehensive reading. To comprehend the texts, literal, inferential, and intertextual questions are asked, the children interact with the text, read in pairs or groups, and finally produce an oral and/or written retelling. Description of the stories: • "Pretty Girl" by Maria Machado is about a dark-skinned girl and her relationship with a white rabbit, who takes a great interest in her because of her skin color and who, in her opinion, makes her the prettiest girl in the world. • "The Tiger and the Mouse" by Keiko Kasza is a story about friendship and how we handle emotions, keeping in mind that it is important to learn to set boundaries for building healthy relationships.
Accompaniment for teachers	Meeting with teachers to agree on the objectives and method of accompaniment. Field diary of the experience of the therapists and the popular educator. Observation and discussion of the photographic record. The teachers' pedagogical practice is captured in photographs that are later used to talk with the teachers about the school routine, the students' play practices, the teaching methodologies, the children's productions.
Discussion with the families	The teachers set up a meeting with the parents of the children in their classes; through play dynamics and questions, the children's daily routines at home are discussed, particularly tasks and the development of habits for their independence in their routines. The families also ask questions and share their concerns about their children.
Inhabiting the territory	Before meeting with the students or teachers, the traditional doctors give a harmonization ceremony as part of the spiritual preparation we must have to get closer to the Indigenous community's education perspective. We also participate in the rituals of fire harmonization, *Sek Buy* and *Inti Raymi*, and awakening of seeds and the XV agroecological market, an event that promotes the sale of locally grown, chemical-free agricultural products, supporting sustainable farming and healthy eating. All this is necessary to feel the territory and to prepare us to work in the community.

Occupational therapy training at the University of Brasília, Faculty of Ceilândia, Brazil

The occupational therapy training program at the University of Brasília, Faculty of Ceilândia, began in 2008. The program, which lasts four years, integrates the preventive, care, and promotional levels of occupational therapy, considering biological and social aspects.

It is important to highlight that the Faculty of Ceilândia and the occupational therapy program emerged from the Support Program toward the

Restructuration Plans and Expansion of Federal Universities, outlined by Decree Nº 6.096 on April 24th, 2007, issued by the Ministry of Education. The purpose of this measure was to broaden people's access to higher education and lower the withdrawal rates of university students. In addition, this measure was made possible due to the demands of social movements in Ceilândia, a peripheral city in the Federal District, advocating for free and public access to universities.

Despite the occupational therapy program's years of experience, students argued that not a single class had addressed issues of race and ethnicity or explored anti-racist practices. Consequently, students joined to protest for a program incorporating these crucial issues. Following student protests in favor of the inclusion of race, ethnicity, and anti-racist practices in occupational therapy training, initiated by a petition organized by Black students, the teachers accepted the changes, and, from this, a subject was created that addresses the specificities of the Black population in terms of their health needs, structural determinants, and historical-social factors.

Their petition was widely circulated among students and the academic center's social media accounts; they collected 105 signatures. The results were shared with the program professors, who gladly agreed to the discussion and proposed the content to be included in the class called Occupational Therapy Inquiry I. Regardless of its name, every term in this class has different topics to discuss, aiming to improve students' education.

Consequently, since 2021, an elective class in "Social Markers of Difference and Anti-Oppressive Praxis," taught by Professor Magno Nunes Farias, has been offered every semester. The course comprehensively addresses the historical and structural aspects of an unequal and contradictory society. It explores social markers of difference, such as status, race/ethnicity, gender, sexuality, generation, disability, and territory, among others, along with oppressive structures and levels of oppression. Additionally, it delves into topics of injustice and social justice, everyday and social transformations, and therapeutic-occupational work in micro-macro-social dialectics. Moreover, it emphasizes therapeutic-occupational anti-oppressive and anti-racist praxis. According to Farias and Lopes (2022), the main idea is to foster a dialogue with a therapeutic-occupational practice that challenges all ways of oppression, viewing occupational therapy as a practice for freedom and against oppression.

The students are highly committed to the class, nurturing their critical thinking skills by engaging in discussions about the diverse experiences of individuals and collectives marked by oppressive logic. They explore how occupational therapy can contribute to their emancipation. One activity that students engage in is the construction of a "self-narrative" (see Figure 3.1), where they explore their social markers of difference. This activity aims to identify how these markers influence their daily lives.

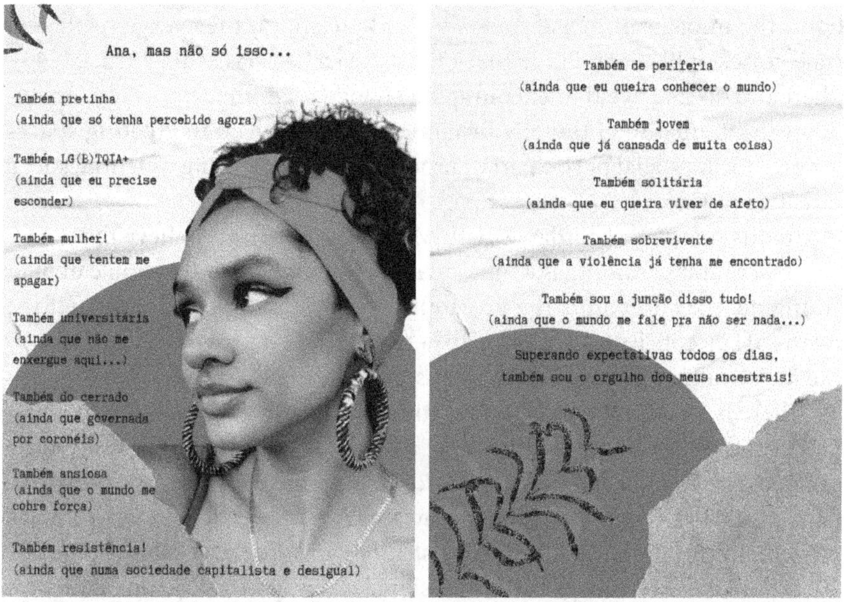
Ana, mas não só isso...
Também pretinha
(ainda que só tenha percebido agora)
Também LG(B)TQIA+
(ainda que eu precise esconder)
Também mulher!
(ainda que tentem me apagar)
Também universitária
(ainda que não me enxergue aqui...)
Também do cerrado
(ainda que governada por coronéis)
Também ansiosa
(ainda que o mundo me cobre força)
Também resistência!
(ainda que numa sociedade capitalista e desigual)
Também de periferia
(ainda que eu queira conhecer o mundo)
Também jovem
(ainda que já cansada de muita coisa)
Também solitária
(ainda que eu queira viver de afeto)
Também sobrevivente
(ainda que a violência já tenha me encontrado)
Também sou a junção disso tudo!
(ainda que o mundo me fale pra não ser nada...)
Superando expectativas todos os dias,
também sou o orgulho dos meus ancestrais!

Figure 3.1 "Self-narrative" activity made by student Ana Laura Gomes de Moura in the Occupational Therapy Inquiry I class from the occupational therapy program at the University of Brasília, Faculty of Ceilândia, in 2021

This experience demonstrates the significance of elective and mandatory classes addressing social markers of difference in occupational therapy programs. These classes challenge a reductionist, uncritical, and biomedical training. Instead, they promote the development of socially committed professionals.

Thus, one of the purposes of this experience is to address the WFOT's emphasis (WFOT, 2010) on the importance of training occupational therapists who are sensitive to topics related to people's contextual diversity and can implement inclusive and socially safe practices.

In addition, the initiative organized by the students resulted in significant transformations in one of the mandatory subjects. The revised version of the subject is still under development. However, once it is ready, it will emphasize the discussion of ethnic-racial concerns and legitimize the training of occupational therapists at the University of Brasília, Faculty of Ceilândia.

Final reflections

Farias et al. (2020) suggest that for occupational therapy to promote social participation, it is essential to understand the racially unequal social structure "starting from the construction of a professional practice that highlights the impacts of racial inequality and racism on the everyday life and trajectories of Black and non-Black individuals" (Farias et al., 2020, p. 243). Therefore, we believe that encouraging change is an important step for students in occupational therapy programs to be involved in creating spaces for promoting social participation processes and discerning potential social transformations.

In this sense, in accordance with Munanga (2005), we believe that occupational therapy training is a fundamental space where "education can offer young people and adults the possibility to question and de-construct the myths of superiority and inferiority between human groups internalized by the racist culture in which they were socialized" (p. 17).

There is an urgent need for education as a practice of freedom for occupational therapy, based on dialogue, awareness, and critical reflection on being in the world (Farias & Lopes, 2022; Freire, 2013), "to implement an education that openly condemns racism. As intellectuals and the Black movement emphasize, education must adopt an anti-racist stance" (Gomes, 2018, p. 14). The challenge that professional training in occupational therapy faces is to incorporate decolonial contents, methodologies, and didactics that establish the ethnic-racial issue as an essential category in the practice of the profession. This not only requires special care to avoid objectifying the experiences of racialized individuals but also entails recognizing them as creators of knowledge, which helps to decentralize our profession from its dominant colonial matrix.

References

Altmann, P. (2016). Buen Vivir como propuesta política integral: Dimensiones del Sumak Kawsay. *Mundos Plurales – Revista Latinoamericana De Políticas Y Acción Pública, 3*(1), 55–74. https://doi.org/10.17141/mundosplurales.1.2016.2318

Ambrosio, L., Riquelme, V., Morrison, R., Gonçalves, A., & Silva, C. (2021). La urgencia de una terapia ocupacional antirracista. *Revista de Estudiantes de Terapia Ocupacional, 8*(1), 1–17.

Ambrosio, L., & Silva, C. R. (2022). Interseccionalidad: Un concepto africano y diaspórico para la terapia ocupacional. *Cadernos Brasileños de Terapia Ocupacional, 30*, e3150. https://doi.org/10.1590/2526-8910.ctoEN241431501

Amorim, S., Martins, S., Leite Junior, J., & Farias, M. (2020). "Asfixias sociais" da população negra e questões para a terapia ocupacional. *Revista Interinstitucional Brasileira de Terapia Ocupacional, 4*(5), 719–733. https://doi.org/10.47222/2526-3544.rbto36144

Ayala Mora, E. (2013). El origen del nombre América Latina y la tradición católica del siglo XIX. *Anuario Colombiano De Historia Social Y De La Cultura, 40*(1), 213–241. https://revistas.unal.edu.co/index.php/achsc/article/view/38769

Barros, D. D. (2002). Loucura na sociedade dogon – República do Mali. *Revista de Terapia Ocupacional da Universidade de São Paulo, 13*(2), 64–70.

Beagan, B., Sibbald, K., Bizzeth, S., & Pride, T. (2022a). Systemic racism in Canadian occupational therapy: A qualitative study with therapists. *Canadian Journal of Occupational Therapy, 89*(1), 51–61. https://doi.org/10.1177/00084174211066676

Beagan, B., Sibbald, K., Pride, T., & Bizzeth, S. (2022b). Experiences of epistemic racism among occupational therapists. *Cadernos Brasileiros de Terapia Ocupacional, 30*, e3211. https://doi.org/10.1590/2526-8910.ctoAO24533211

Bezerra, J. B., & Alves, H. C. (2022). Na EKO na EBA – o vai e vem da imigração: Cotidiano, identidade e demandas de imigrantes africanos estudantes universitários. *Cadernos Brasileiros de Terapia Ocupacional, 30*(spe), e3073. https://doi.org/10.1590/2526-8910.ctoAO232630731

Castro, E. D. de, & Lima, E. M. F. de A. (2007). Resistência, inovação e clínica no pensar e no agir de Nise da Silveira. *Interface (Botucatu), 11*(22). https://doi.org/10.1590/S1414-32832007000200017

Costa, M., Santos, A., Souza, J., Costa, J., Porto, R., & Freire, S. (2020). Laboratório Iṣẹ̣: Construções de estratégias para restituição histórica e existêncial de pessoas negras. *Revista Interinstitucional Brasileira de Terapia Ocupacional, 4*(5), 734–741. https://doi.org/10.47222/2526-3544.rbto36913

Cruz, T., Barradas, J., & Sampaio, E. (2021). Infâncias negras de uma comunidade periférica e os significados de ocupar-se do projeto social Afrocine. *Revista Interinstitucional Brasileira de Terapia Ocupacional, 5*(4), 502–519. https://doi.org/10.47222/2526-3544.rbto40821

Defensoría del Pueblo (2019, October 15). Día Nacional de las Personas con Discapacidad. Defensoría del Pueblo Bolivia. www.defensoria.gob.bo/noticias/dia-nacional-de-las-personas-con-discapacidad

Farias, M. N., Leite, J. D., & Amorim, S. G. S. (2020). Para la formación y la práctica antirracista: Consideraciones para la terapia ocupacional. *Revista Chilena De Terapia Ocupacional, 20*(2), 237–247. https://doi.org/10.5354/0719-5346.2020.54658

Farias, M., Leite, J., & Costa, I. (2018). Terapia ocupacional e população negra: Possibilidades para o enfrentamento do racismo e desigualdade racial. *Revista Interinstitucional Brasileira de Terapia Ocupacional, 2*(1), 228–243. https://doi.org/10.47222/2526-3544.rbto12712

Farias, M. N., & Lopes, R. E. (2022). Terapia ocupacional social, antiopressão e liberdade: Considerações sobre a revolução da/na vida cotidiana. *Cadernos Brasileiros de Terapia Ocupacional, 30*(spe), e3100. https://doi.org/10.1590/2526-8910.ctoEN234531002

Farias, M., & Vicente, H. (2022). Debatendo o racismo na universidade: Ação prática da terapia ocupacional e psicologia. *Revista Interinstitucional Brasileira de Terapia Ocupacional, 6*(1), 815–821. https://doi.org/10.47222/2526-3544.rbto39265

Fernandes, P. F. A. L., Andreade, A. F., Ambrosio, L., & Fragelli, C. (2021). "É som de preto, de favelado": O funk como forma de (r)existência para crianças e adolescentes em acolhimento. *Revista Interinstitucional Brasileira de Terapia Ocupacional, 4*(5), 632–638. https://doi.org/10.47222/2526-3544.rbto41463

França, M. M. L., Queiroz, S. B., & Bezerra, W. C. (2016). Saúde dos povos de terreiro, práticas de cuidado e terapia ocupacional: Um diálogo possível? *Cadernos Brasileiros de Terapia Ocupacional, 24*(1), 105–116.

Freire, P. (2013). *À Sombra desta Mangueira.* Rio de Janeiro: Paz e Terra.

Fuentes, J. A., Linfati, F. S., Opazo, M. A., Rodríguez, V. P., & Reyes, V. E. (2020). Impacto de la violencia política en el juego de niños y niñas Mapuche de una comunidad de la Región de la Araucanía. *Revista Chilena De Terapia Ocupacional, 20*(1), 73–82. https://doi.org/10.5354/0719-5346.2020.51355

Gomes, N. L. (2018). Apresentação. In P. V. B. Silva, K. Regias, & S. A. Miranda (Eds.), *Educação das Relações Étnico-raciais: O Estado da Arte.* Curitiba: NEAB-UFPR; ABPN.

Gomez Correal, D. (2020). Améfrica Ladina, Abya Yala y nuestra América: Tejiendo esperanzas realistas. *LASA Forum*, pp. 55–59.

Hopenhayn, M., & Bello, A. (2001). *Discriminación Étnico-racial y Xenofobia en América Latina y el Caribe.* Santiago: United Nations.

Leite, J. D., Farias, M. N., & Martins, S. (2021). Dona Ivone Lara e terapia ocupacional: Devir-negro da história da profissão. *Cadernos Brasileiros de Terapia Ocupacional, 29*, e2171. https://doi.org/10.1590/2526-8910.ctoARF2171

Leite, P., de Andrade, A., Ambrosio, L., & Fragelli, C. (2021). "É som de preto, de favelado": O funk como forma de (r)existência para crianças e adolescentes em acolhimento. *Revista Interinstitucional Brasileira de Terapia Ocupacional, 5*(4), 632–638. https://doi.org/10.47222/2526-3544.rbto41463

Lozano Lerma, B. R. (2019). *Aportes a un Feminismo Negro Decolonial: Insurgencias Epistémicas de Mujeresnegras-Afrocolombianas Tejidas con Retazos de Memoria: Vol. 1*. Editorial Abya-Yala.

Macedo, M. D., Teresa de Lima Neves, A., Bardi, G., Monzeli, G. A., & Mota, V. V. (2016). Olhares em formação: Refletindo a prática da terapia ocupacional em um contexto cultural a partir de experiências com povos indígenas. *Cadernos Brasileiros De Terapia Ocupacional, 24*(1), 77–89. https://doi.org/10.4322/0104-4931.ctoAO0665

Munanga, K. (2005). Apresentação. In K. Munanga (Ed.), *Superando o Racismo na Escola*. Brasília: Ministério da Educação, Secretaria de Educação Continuada, Alfabetização e Diversidade.

Pastore, M. D. N., & Sato, M. T. (2018). Pelos caminhos da diversidade sociocultural: Diálogos entre terapia ocupacional, África e etnografia. *Cadernos Brasileiros De Terapia Ocupacional, 26*(4), 952–959. https://doi.org/10.4322/2526-8910.ctoARF1240

Pérez, C., Nazar, G., & Cova, F. (2016). Facilitadores y obstaculizadores de la implementación de la política de salud intercultural en Chile. *Revista Panamericana de Salud Pública, 39*(2), 122–127. www.scielosp.org/article/rpsp/2016.v39n2/122-127

Perilla, V. M. L., Magalhães, L., Pérez, D. K. C., Olivero, M. M. A., et al. (2021). "O bicho, aquele pirralho" nos territórios indígenas colombianos: Tecendo diálogos com a comunidade Kankuama em tempos de pandemia. *Cadernos Brasileiros de Terapia Ocupacional, 29*, e2836. https://doi.org/10.1590/2526-8910.ctoAO2146

Rojas, C. P. (2017). Terapia ocupacional en el post acuerdo: Retos para una profesión que se transforma. *Revista Ocupación Humana, 17*(1), 3–6. https://doi.org/10.25214/25907816.150

Universidad Andrés Bello. (2017). *Aprueba el Nuevo Plan de Estudios de la Carrera de Terapia Ocupacional*, DUN° 2497/2017. Santiago.

Universidad Mayor de San Andrés. (2019). *Informe de Autoevaluación de los Programas de Terapia Ocupacional y Fonoaudiologia. Propuesta Carrera de Ciencias de la Rehabilitación*. Editorial WAGUI. La Paz, Bolivia.

Valério, A. C. O., Bezerra, W. C., Santos, V. S., Leite, J. D., Farias, M. N., & Santos, S. M. B. (2021). Racismo e participação social na universidade: Experiências de estudantes negras em cursos de saúde. *Cadernos Brasileiros de Terapia Ocupacional, 29*, e3007. https://doi.org/10.1590/2526-8910.ctoAO2278

Vigoya, M. V. (2021). Los colores del antirracismo (en Améfrica Ladina). *Sexualidad, Salud y Sociedad* (Rio de Janeiro), no. 36, 19–34. https://doi.org/10.1590/1984-6487.sess.2020.36.02.a

WFOT. (2010). *Position Statement on Diversity and Culture*. World Federation of Occupational Therapy. https://wfot.org/about/wfot-statements

CHAPTER 4

Autobiographical Writing and Other Places of Resistance in Occupational Therapy

IDENTITIES AND PRAXIS FROM THE SOUTH

Aída del Pilar Becerra Becerra, Yenny Patricia López Díaz, and Iara Falleiros Braga

Abstract

The theme of identity suggests plural, intersubjective, and intercultural exploration. This chapter presents the reflections of three Latin American women, occupational therapists, and graduates of public academic institutions in Brazil, Colombia, and Spain. For nine months, the authors shared their reflections orally and via virtual media, using autobiography as both a means and an end in their writing. Each section registers ways of living and transmitting occupational therapy practice based on experiences and discourses that inevitably emerge from places of resistance. In the first part of this chapter, a thematic framework for what constitutes autobiographical writing is developed. The following three sections convey identities through the authors' narratives. These identities are then articulated in the fifth and final section, which weaves intersectionalities using decolonial perspectives. This chapter is an invitation to cultivate a deeper understanding of the evolving landscape of occupational therapy by highlighting perspectives, experiences, and identities that challenge established norms, provoke critical thought, and encourage innovative approaches to knowledge construction and professional practice within the field.

Keywords

occupational therapy; identity; praxis; autobiography; resistance

Learning outcomes

- Analyze critical and counter-hegemonic perspectives in occupational therapy, illustrating alternative avenues for knowledge and practice construction and dissemination within the profession.
- Value personal and professional experiences embodying the challenges the evolving occupational therapy profession faces across social, health, educational, community, research, academic, personal, local, and global domains.
- Discuss a methodological approach for creating historically contextualized texts in occupational therapy, demonstrating a commitment to social engagement and understanding the personal, professional, and societal transformations demanded by contemporary times.
- Foster a deeper comprehension of the field's dynamic evolution and encourage critical thinking and innovation in knowledge construction and professional development through exposure to diverse viewpoints and experiences within occupational therapy.

Introduction: Voices and glances to create with six hands

The consequences of the COVID-19 pandemic, political, social, and military conflicts, environmental problems, and climate change have colored contemporary times, revealing the inexorable transformation of the habitual. Thus, thinking about identities and occupational therapy practices from the South draws attention to paradigm shifts that transcend and break conceptions, allowing for new perspectives on reality (Gergen, 2006, 2016, and Taylor, 2006, in López, 2019). In this context, we refer to identities as dynamic features associated with one's own experience but also as opportunities for encounter and consensus between discourses, practices, and subjectivizing processes (Hall, 2003, in López, 2019).

In this chapter, the deconstruction of autobiographical narratives became a means of acknowledging the existence not only of the individual but also of collective subjects, which have historically been conditioned by concurrent sociopolitical, economic, and cultural realities (Garcia-Ruiz, 2016; Núñez, 2019; Simó, 2016). In this sense, professional practices indicate the existence of different epistemologies emerging from the Global South to nourish new identities and praxis[1] from intersectional voices and viewpoints. Intersec-

1 Within occupational therapy, praxis is defined as the process of articulating reflection and action for social transformation, that is, for the emancipation of individuals and collectives, to ensure respect for diversity and social justice (Galheigo, 2012).

tionality is "an approach that, within the framework of modernity/coloniality's effects in different spaces and times in Latin America, allows us to address the link between difference and power" (Sória, 2023, p. 13). Thus, intersectional voices and perspectives recognize resistance spaces where oppressive structures perpetuating racism, classism, and other forms of injustice and violence can be challenged.

The methodological approach of this chapter is founded on identification, trust, orality, and listening. It contains a variety of views and voices that come together in the re-signification and re-appropriation of at least three identities: authors, narrators, and characters (Lejeune, 1991). On this premise, and for nine months, we established a virtual *circle of words*[2] in which we discussed autobiographical writing as a place of resistance and its relationship to occupational therapy identities and praxis from the South. In addition, to widen our viewpoints, we asked nine female readers (three for each author) to read our rough writings as occupational biographers.[3]

With this in mind, the first autobiographical text examines alternative occupational therapy practices via the lens of situated being and doing; the second explores life paths in which the author sees limitations as opportunities for action and transformation; and the final section examines the aspects that reverberate in a collective and transformative practice.

Contributions on being and doing: An autobiographical text by Aída del Pilar Becerra

I am an artist, occupational therapist, and social researcher who likes listening, writing, and weaving stories. I am part of a semi-nomadic and intercultural family that transits between continents. My work combines research and creative experiences in community, education, and mental health with a differential and rights-based approach. I am moved by life's transformative capacity revealed through birds, waves, and communities,

2 Translated from the Spanish *circulo de palabra*, also known as talking circle, owned by First Peoples. The circle of words is defined as a collaborative participation space centered on listening, orality, and silence, in which each member takes turns sharing thoughts through a measured and halted use of the word. Cosmovisions, uses, practices, and individual and community aspects are inherent in the circle.

3 We define occupational biographers as persons who connect with the autobiographical texts from their lived experiences and reflections, occupying biographical spaces from three different perspectives: (a) those who exercise as occupational therapists or who do not, (b) those who are native to Latin America or who are not, and (c) those who have shared our life history or who have not.

through everything that exists. The wise *Mamu*[4] from the Sierra Nevada de Santa Marta, on the northern coast of Colombia (see Figure 4.1), says that as humanity, we will advance when we learn to connect with this movement, to listen to the voice of nature/mother, which speaks through the territories, the plants, and the animals, which in sum are one.

Reflecting with a decolonial perspective, I bring to my thoughts the Asian, European, and American cultures and territories that have welcomed me in which I have lived. I open this writing space with gratitude for the opportunity to travel and get to know other ways of feeling and thinking. Considering the responsibility of speaking from the South,[5] I turn to my history and the teachings of those who have taught me to rethink identities and praxis, being and doing, to present reflections as an autobiographical account.

When the being speaks in the situated doing

A traveling impulse in me has led me to travel the world and approach issues such as ethno-education, bilingualism, and interculturality. I will focus on narrating some of the lessons I have learned from two South American cultures, Cofán and Arhuaca, as a mestizo, taking part in everyday and sacred spaces (see Figure 4.1).

I learned that thinking, speaking, and doing must be linked to manifest balance. The world's knowledge, the great library of wisdom, is nature. Thought comes to life while walking, cooking, weaving, building, or loving; it expresses itself through actions and without words. Thought forges being, and this speaks through doing. Its order or balance is based on the *Law of Origin* or fundamental mandate inscribed in the visible and invisible, reflecting other worlds' existence and their interconnection with the territories that unite them (UNESCO, 2023).

When thought becomes a word, it creates. What is said has value and power. Through oral tradition, communities in general, specifically *knowledgeable men and women,*[6] learn from their families' and teachers' observation and guidance, the laws and mandates of origin guiding individual and

---

4 *Mamu*, also known as *mama* or *mamo*, are the spiritual leaders of the Wintukua people in the Sierra Nevada de Santa Marta in Colombia. They are priests, guides, and counselors. They are community leaders, but they have no political power and possess different specializations and ranks depending on their place of origin, community, lineage, preparation, and religious prestige, among other social identities (Reiter, 2016).

5 I specifically refer to words of life or teachings of the Indigenous peoples that I have had the opportunity to know. To broaden these experiences, visit www.aguamaestra.com

6 Among Indigenous peoples, these individuals develop the necessary abilities and sensitivity to converse with snow-capped peaks, connect with river wisdom, and comprehend nature's messages (UNESCO, 2023).

collective actions. From there, guided by master plants and sacred places, they accompany the physical, mental, and spiritual health of their families, communities, and territories. They are taught to listen to their bodies, dreams, birds, water, plants, and nature, which constitutes the voice of their common mother: the territories, the planet, Mother Earth. Listening is a means of learning to think and speak *bonito* (pretty), which in the deepest sense implies expressing oneself with clarity and respect, ordering one's being and doing, and taking charge of the consequences of what one thinks, says, and does, which is both a vital key and a challenge.

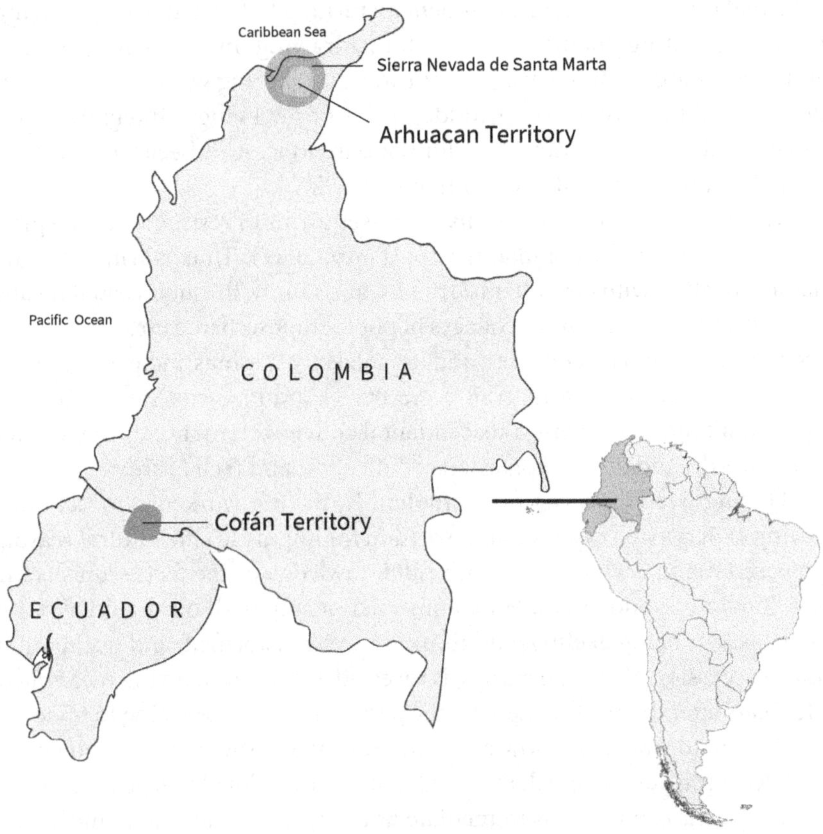

Figure 4.1 Situating the Cofán and Arhuaca cultures in the Sierra Nevada de Santa Marta (made by Pamela Talero)

When doing transforms being

Updating occupational therapy training and practice scenarios implies acknowledging the multiplicity of readings, contexts, histories, and worldviews that converge there. To communicate through doing, we must turn our eyes to the quotidian (everyday), pause, feel, observe, listen, and recognize it as unique, memorable, and even sacred. As a common ground to expand on these statements, I will shortly share aspects of my praxis during the COVID-19 pandemic.

I was in Bogotá, Colombia's capital, my home city. I had lived away from my family and done mostly voluntary telework for nearly ten years, and I was a regular user of digital applications and electronic devices. However, like millions of people across the globe, I was impacted by social isolation and alienation from my loved ones. I understood that I had to take the pieces of the puzzle of my life and create new rules for the game. I returned to virtual therapeutic accompaniment by turning to the living arts, weaving, literature, writing, meditation, breathing, drawing, music, dance, singing, and agroecology. Empowering what I was and sharing what I knew how to do, I brought together lost or hidden parts of my being. I integrated what I liked to do into my praxis but did not dare to show it because it was not formally part of my profession. I freed myself.

The enjoyment of occupations expresses forms of resistance to the pressures imposed by the colonial matrix (Pérez, 2021). Thus, during the pandemic, together with consultants, friends, and family, through virtual means, to resist and re-exist, I made collages of photographs, shared creative cooking sessions, improvised serenades, and organized gatherings and get-togethers. The creative power of arts, crafts, and trades did its own thing, conjuring up difficult moments with transcendental conversations, bursts of laughter, sweet words, and other expressions of affection and (self) care.

Having lived far away from my family, having worked remotely, and having experienced distance and isolation for linguistic and cultural reasons prepared me to accompany—with full knowledge of the facts—uncertainties, loneliness, and crises. When our relationship with our habitual doing changes, our being, feeling, and thinking are transformed, and occupation, as an expression of human beings, is revealed as the key to giving meaning to life. Years after the confinement by the pandemic, it is interesting to review—in addition to where and how it is communicated—the scope we can give to such learning beyond borders. As inhabitants of a global village of the same planet, praxis can allow us to mediate not only in the balance of individual occupational performance but also in social justice and peace for humanity.

Biocartography: A technique to map being and doing

I propose biocartography as a technique for collecting and analyzing qualitative information that explores biographical occupational aspects (moments) and cartographic aspects (places). It combines the writing of logs (by periods, events, quadrenniums, septenniums) and the drawing of maps (bodily, geographical, fantastic, networks). It requires exercises or practices that can be projected into the present, past, and future with poetic writings, photographs, images, and sounds, among other resources. It is a means of self-observation, listening to one's voice, re-signifying experiences, and broadening the horizon of knowledge and action. With texts from my logs, I will exemplify possibilities for applying this technique of tracing, exploration, and occupational expression in development.

Starting a Biocartography: Guidelines

Tracing

Place on a timeline places and dates (in the example, every four years) accompanied by a phrase that synthesizes a representative memory of the moments of the life cycle that you identify as milestones (crises, achievements, closures, etc.).

Example:

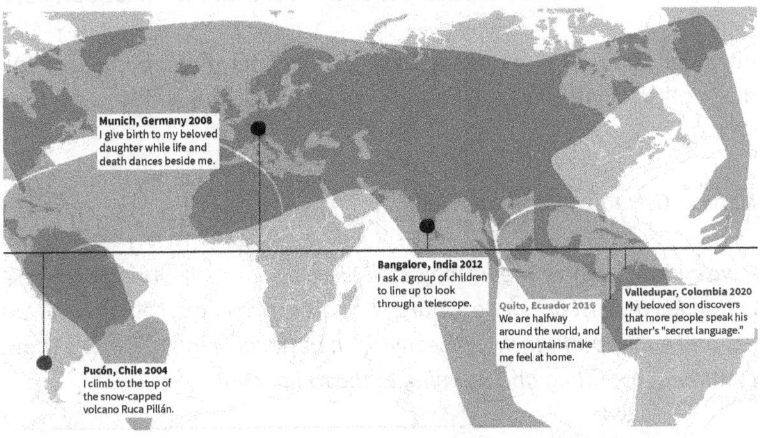

Figure 4.2 Example of a timeline for recording and representing experiences (made by Pamela Talero)

Note that the pattern for your timeline can: (a) be carried out with other, not necessarily regular, time cycles; (b) invite the consultee to record information in code; (c) be recorded on geographical, body, or support network maps; (d) include symbolic, representative elements, photographs, songs, or emblematic phrases, among other descriptions; (e) make in/direct reference to people, places, and situations; and (f) be extended to dates, audiovisual, narrative, or pictorial explorations, and reduced with icons next to the place and year marked.

Exploring

In this stage, you will explore significant moments and places through narrative. Photographs may accompany it. Experiences, lessons learned, and socio-occupational adaptations can be traced for occupational exploration or psychosocial accompaniment. Contrast challenging experiences and experiences that have shown you new perspectives.

Example:

Bogotá, Colombia, July 2001

As a degree option, we created an occupational therapy program, VIHDA, for people diagnosed with HIV/AIDS, taking up the Colombian Model of "fulfilling Occupational Performance" (Castillo Aguas & Varón Caicedo, 2017). We included activities for each dimension: Autonomy, Socialization, Productivity, and Achievement, grounded in the social and family context. We converged in spaces of trust for listening and workshops in which what made each participant unique (personality, histories, qualities, beliefs, and expectations) configured the navigation chart of their therapeutic process.

Although the narrative above is part of my personal records, the full description of VIHDA can be found in Becerra-Becerra and Moreno-Sosa (2003).

Munich, Germany, December 2005

It was my first winter in Germany. I felt like a conch shell. During the week, I attended at least one open lecture and visited museums, churches, libraries, and public parks to immerse myself in the local language. In the snow, I returned to knitting and listening to the radio.

I used this metaphor that refers to people who carry their homes on their tails in the chapter I titled "Traveling sea snails: Violence, occupational changes, and migrant women" (Becerra-Becerra, 2011).

Munich, Germany, January 2009

We created the GalileoMobile! Project. This experience of popularizing science took me to South American and Indian schools.

To know more, visit www.galileomobile.org/audiovisuals

Biocartography, as a developing technique, is an invitation to create grounded, situated, and historicized roadmaps that provide individuals, families, and even organizations with inputs to review what they need to decant, purify, or order. Nowadays, various technological and computer programming tools allow for qualitative and quantitative information[7] analysis that can broaden its scope. This tool facilitates the communication of experiences and learning about being and doing. Events that involve closing and opening cycles, such as a professional achievement, a journey, or a health event, allow us to trace the characteristics of contexts, cultures, territories, and other scenarios of being and doing. Applying this filter of analysis and translating it not only into words but also into drawings, symbols, and images gives depth to the therapeutic process. It is pedagogical insofar as it makes it meaningful and receptive.

I encourage us to continue reflecting on the dialectical and transformative potential of doing and to develop or use complementary tools to praxis without fearing breaks or ruptures in interpreting reality. We are on the right track if they bring joy, calm, happiness, security, confidence, or well-being to balance our being and doing. At this point, every place, date, and experience, from the everyday to the sacred, appear as opportunities to trace routes ever closer to what we want to be and do. There are as many pages to be written and routes to be traveled as each being decides to take.

A (self-)critical and decolonial gaze is a provocation to make other occupational therapies visible: An autobiographical text by Yenny P. López Díaz

Inspired by Rodó-Zárate (2021), I recognize that my perspective is inherently situated and partial, shaped by my positionality and the context in which I navigate.

I write to offer reading prisms of what could be called cartography of my professional work from the categories of woman, Colombian, childless, and immigrant, among others. The text seeks to make visible the coordinates of the different axes of inequality between what it means to be an occupational therapist and to do occupational therapy in the different territories I have inhabited and the contexts I have lived in.

My story talks about the normative mechanisms I have experienced in the last 20 years, both in Colombia and Spain, concerning what occupational therapists do. The experience of individuals acting from the occupational

7 Product of autobiographical texts, diagramming frequencies of words that refer to places, people, situations, ties, emotions, and qualifiers, among other categories.

therapist role can be understood via intersectionality dynamics (Rodó-Zárate, 2021). A professional profile is typically expected to conform to normative expectations following globally structured academic frameworks that have historically exhibited colonial characteristics (Freire, 1970). These frameworks are often influenced by imaginaries rooted in productivity-oriented ideals.

In counterpoint to these mechanisms, other ways of doing and occupying what we do with organic and sustainable practices for life are emerging from the South (López Díaz, 2015). I am intrigued as to how we make these ways of doing occupational therapy visible and, above all, how we legitimize them within the academic and professional structure. One way of doing so invites us to visit places within and outside the academy, to listen and talk to other divergent and dissenting voices, to walk other occupational paths than the legitimized ones, and to make known other possibilities in the practice of our profession (Silvestrini, Silva, & Prado, 2019; Turcotte & Holmes, 2021).

Discussing our professional identities and how they are transformed and altered by the territories we inhabit is critical. Whether these practices need to be legitimized, regulated, regularized, and systematized is debatable. Spaces both inside and outside of academia, such as professional associations and colleges of occupational therapy, can serve as innovation laboratories and weave networks with other disciplines to make known and strengthen the diversity of our professional practices. Professional practice embodies what we do and who we are when we do it. Sharing this experience has the intimate feel of autobiographical writing and is a good starting point for approaching the diversity of "ways of doing" occupational therapy. This motivates me to embark on an autobiographical journey tracing crucial components in my historicity to feel and think about the intersectional dynamics that shape the making of my occupation. I hope they can inspire or motivate you to tell your story.

First stop: The (auto)biographical glance

Cantero Garlito et al. (2012) argued that "occupational therapists have paid little attention to sex. Even gender [...]. It is surprising that [...] in a profession with an overwhelming majority of women, occupational therapy has never had a feminist ideology" (p. 99). This comment, which contrasts with reflections from colleagues and friends in Colombia, made me consider the incredible ignorance of feminist practices in occupational therapy. Moreover, they led me to admit that the question of gender and macho violence were issues that took me a long time to address. I had to write a doctoral thesis on the autobiographies of Colombian and Spanish teachers (López, 2019) to delve into the mechanisms of violence and, in addition, I had to recognize myself as a victim and victimizer within the dynamics of inequality between categories such as Latin American-immigrant-woman (Butler, 2004, 2006).

An autobiography does not need to be accompanied by the word *occupational* to be autobiographical because it is the narration of one's life (Lejeune, 1991). We usually narrate a life in facts or actions within a timeline. When we write our autobiography, we remember moments that are milestones or identity markers. Personal identity is the possibilities of action that the subject can take within a timeline of conditionings; these can be enabling or constraining. This characteristic can be extrapolated to professional identity, since professions are sets of actions shared by communities. Each autobiographical exercise represents a point of existence that reveals an identity position. In this way, each autobiography could be interpreted as a reflection, a beam of light, or a trace of identity.

The autobiographies of those of us who play the role of occupational therapists are reflections of the multiplicity of ways of doing occupational therapy, and recognizing this multiplicity is the organic way of synchronizing ourselves with the realities and territories in which we live. These autobiographical lines express my existence through a fluid image of myself. Here, I expose myself and the conditions that make me be and shape my work as an occupational therapy practitioner. They contain the traces that I leave on my path and intend to expose my feelings and actions as a holobiont that moves through its intersections.

The intersectionality that runs through me

My practice as a professional does not escape this act of reflection. On several occasions, I have found myself in places where the patriarchal hierarchy anchored in hegemonic narratives develops imaginaries that determine what a person trained in the occupational therapy profession is expected to do. These imaginaries delimit and limit the possibilities of exercising a more organic and sustainable practice.

When I finished my undergraduate studies in Colombia, I was faced with the reality of a flexible labor market and the absence of a welfare and social protection system. I understood then that there were spaces reserved for professions and that the one I chose had the space of care reserved for it. Of course, a feminized profession was to be found among the paramedical professions, parallel to the medical professions as satellites. Then, within these satellites, you find professions with a better known and more highly valued career. I experienced how occupational therapists were constantly challenged to justify our field of action to avoid invading other professional spaces. Now, I see that entering other territories of human activity is inevitable, as this is our profession's meaning.

Throughout my professional trajectory, I remember feeling the weight of having to be a "good" therapist, a perception intimately related to the idea of being a "good" woman. From my life story, and maybe yours too, the territory for occupational therapy practices is delimited by a bias that burdens the profession with care-related tasks. Tasks in a cis-hetero-patriarchal society come from the private sphere (Arendt, 2005; Birulés, 2015) and are imposed and associated with being a woman. Today, I see how these conditioning factors have marked my experiences and, to a large extent, my occupational opportunities.

The burden of the duty led me to consider that my professional possibilities have been limited, bound, and objectified by gender biases that, like invisible barriers, instrumentalize our work. Thinking about the concept of a "good" therapist carrying the cultural burden of the idea of a "good woman," I admit that this quality varies in territory and time. However, I consider that there are shared impressions and experiences, such as considering ourselves responsible for improving a person in our care. Caregiving is the ultimate task we acquire as therapists, especially from a health perspective. It is so ingrained in our practices that we consider it the third part of any human being's occupational performance.

Added to these conditions is the idea of a globalized occupational therapist profile that fits like a joker in any context. This worries me because hegemonic ideas about occupational therapy practice appear to me as a significant threat of oppression with a colonial heritage that erases ancestral practices and drags them into oblivion. I recognize the importance of generating shared knowledge through conceptual structures that allow us to identify the multiplicity of practices. Global indicators and standards for both the training of professionals and the practice of the profession are primarily necessary to assess our processes. However, considering these parameters as rules instead of collective agreements leads to approaches that classify, reduce, and limit occupational practices and opportunities, which are reactionary to social changes and cultural transformations. Hence the call to continue unveiling these limiting ideas and stereotypical behaviors as a learning community and to self-criticism of our professional identity, an exercise we must undertake to face the current challenges.

My resistance to fitting in and inhabiting the margin

I emigrated more than a decade ago. As a Latin American immigrant in Spain, my working life in Colombia is not formally recognized, meaning that everything I did before coming here belongs to another world. This condition of oblivion has forced me to delve into other places I had not explored in Colombia, such as community culture. Here in Spain, I have participated in community spaces such as Harinera ZGZ,[8] where I have found other ways to practice as an occupational therapist, freeing myself from labels that tie me to social and healthcare spaces with rehabilitative perspectives. In these places, I have collectively created projects that promote people's well-being by creating social and community fabric, using art and creativity as a means of expression.

When I emigrated, I passed my occupational therapy practice through the sieve. The delicate parts were separated from the coarse ones because, as I had no work history, social fabric, or academic ties to sustain me, my occupational opportunities were scarce and were marked, as I mentioned a few lines back, by stereotypical gender dynamics that materialized in the territory of care,[9] leaving the feminization of the profession (Freire de Araújo & Lima de Paula, 2023; Mora Augier, 2022) exposed. I would add the condition of immigrants, foreigners, and Latin Americans.

Recognizing the dynamics of inequality and oppression within our training and professional practices has been fundamental. For this, autobiographical exercises have been of immense value as reflective acts to reinterpret my story from the affection and care of myself. This is an invitation to the autobiographical exercise to transfigure our doings, to turn around what we take for granted from our theoretical models as the meaning of occupation and purpose of occupational performance. In my writing exercises, I have found that my professional practice is not recognized within the established limits; it is a practice that struggles to transform limiting conditions and to rewrite from the condition of "foreigner," ideas of individualization that place me in the territory of competitiveness and not of solidarity and collaboration. Thus, I recognize my taste for inhabiting the margin, not in separation or isolation but as an explorer who transits through territories.

Living on the margins has been a constant since I was very young. With every migration I made, I perceived it. Living on the margins does not mean I do not live with intensity. On the contrary, being there permits you to be awake and engage with your present to identify the keys that allow you to participate in the community.

By inhabiting the margin, actions can be extended to other places, which makes it easier to move through the territories. Migration is, therefore, an enabling condition. Migration as movement is the trace that allows us to recognize the journey, the path of existence. My mother migrated several times, and we went with her; we migrated from one neighborhood to another

8 You can learn more about community spaces such as Harinera ZGZ at https://reacc.org
9 Care is understood as a set of actions that correspond to people's intimate lives and have been taken into the public sphere throughout history due to the need to maintain a social and economic structure based on patriarchy (Birulés, 2015).

and from one school to another. We migrated from the city and territory. We migrated affections and customs. I migrated from the country. I migrated from work. In short, migrating is a category sheltered within my condition as a foreigner. Recognizing this condition makes it easier for me to connect with the diversity of realities and enabling and limiting conditions within which I live. Moreover, with this, I recognize other ways of doing occupational therapy that allow me to address social needs through solidarity and cooperation in favor of a fairer world.

Activity: Inhabiting the Margin

Think about your journey as a member of the occupational therapy profession and how the social categories that characterize you have shaped this journey. What limits or margins have you or anyone else set for yourself and others?

Having reflected on the limits or margins, debate your agreement or dissent with the following:

Why inhabit the margin?

By inhabiting it, you are considered a foreigner, which allows you not to be inside the whole and, at the same time, not to be part of that whole, keeping the proper distance to act. From this place, other forms of occupational therapy that are more organic and sustainable can emerge.

How do you inhabit the margin?

When I participate in a community, I abandon the idea of being the savior, as special or efficient. I go with a humble attitude of collaborating and weaving. I intend to give what the community needs from me, which is often far from what I think they need. Observing what a community requires is the first step in opening new ways of doing and allowing those realities to emerge that are enriched by our actions.

Movements in action and transformation: Reflections on the production of knowledge and the practice of occupational therapies: An autobiographical text by Iara Falleiros Braga

Drawing from Bondía (2002), I recognize that truly experiencing something requires an intentional pause—an interruption from the fast pace of daily life. It calls for slowing down our thinking, observing with care, listening attentively, and allowing ourselves to feel deeply. It means suspending immediate judgment, stepping away from automatic responses, and instead cultivating patience, openness, and a sensitivity to the details that shape our understanding.

I begin this autobiographical account by reflecting on my own experience—not as an isolated narrative, but as one that is both personal and shared. My identity has been shaped through a tapestry of moments, encounters, and collective knowledge, woven together like a patchwork of intersecting stories that continue to evolve.

To situate my professional and personal experience, it is also necessary to reflect on the sociohistorical reality of Brazil, a country with an intense production of social inequality. Brazil is a country with great cultural diversity, wealth, and natural beauty. However, it bears the marks of colonialism, with a racist, sexist, fascist, and LGBTQ-phobic structure that daily exterminates and exploits the Indigenous population, *quilombolas*,[10] and other traditional communities. This has increased the concentration of income and poverty that massively imprisons mainly poor and Black youth, which has a prominent upward movement of political conservatism with severe threats to democracy (Braga *et al.*, 2020).

Traditional peoples and communities are culturally differentiated groups that are recognized as such, that have their forms of social organization, that occupy and use territories and natural resources as a condition for their cultural, social, religious, ancestral, and economic reproduction, using knowledge, innovations, and practices generated and transmitted by tradition (Brazilian Government, 2007). These groups include Indigenous peoples, *quilombolas*, river dwellers, rubber tappers, artisanal fishermen, and family farmers. The groups have in common the struggle to recognize their rights, preserve their traditions and ways of life, and protect their lands and natural resources. The Brazilian Constitution[11] recognizes their rights and their vital role in preserving the country's cultural and environmental diversity; nevertheless, the deterritorialization of traditional peoples and communities is a violation practiced since colonization.

Faced with so many threats and such a complex structure of society, in 2004 I began my career in occupational therapy, mobilized to understand,

10 Predominantly Black ethnic groups, found throughout the Brazilian territory, identifiable according to a category of self-attribution commonly designated as "lands of black people." The term *quilombola* is used to describe the inhabitants of these communities, who continue to preserve their cultural and historical heritage, contributing to the ethnic and cultural diversity of Brazil (de Figueiredo, 2011).

11 Constituição da República Federativa do Brasil de 1988: www.planalto.gov.br/ccivil_03/constituicao/constituicao.htm

study, research, and technically appropriate occupational therapy as a powerful profession for transforming social reality. Thus, in the second year at occupational therapy school, I joined the Metuia UFSCar[12] laboratory, where I could experience teaching, research, and outreach activities in social occupational therapy.

Social occupational therapy is a theoretical area of occupational therapy developed in Brazil, with its own theoretical and methodological framework in search of the emancipation and autonomy of subjects with socioeconomic impediments and difficulties in accessing their social rights. It focuses on the individual and collective subjects, emphasizing their social position and the possibilities in their daily lives, understanding the occupational therapist as capable of generating joint strategies to expand opportunities (Malfitano, 2016).

Thus, social occupational therapy bases and creates its theoretical and methodological foundations on the objective of social justice, more dignified living conditions, and access to social rights (Galheigo et al., 2018), with its referents, methods, and techniques, understanding that the health-related theory and methodological referents and contributions are not able to respond to the specific demands of the social field.

In this laboratory, I developed actions at the micro- and macrosocial level, mainly aimed at poor and peripheral young people in São Carlos. We articulated territorial actions involving various teams of the social support network, such as the school, the youth center, and the social assistance reference center, among other spaces, in addition to carrying out a workshop on activities, dynamics, and projects, singular and territorial accompaniments, and the Articulation of Resources in the Social Field and Dynamization of the Service Network—which are social technologies aimed at strengthening support networks (Lopes et al., 2014).

I frequently worked with young people facing social vulnerability, a condition shaped by the intersection of precarious employment and weak social ties. This reality affects a significant portion of the Brazilian population, highlighting systemic challenges. Factors such as extreme inequality, migration to large urban centers, inadequate housing, and the historical structure of the Brazilian nuclear family—combined with widespread labor

12 The Metuia Network was created in 1998 by professors of the undergraduate courses in occupational therapy of the Federal University of São Carlos (UFSCar), the University of Sao Paulo (USP), and the Pontifical Catholic University of Campinas (PUC-Campinas), aiming to institutionalize and develop research, training, and practices around occupational associate therapy, focusing on issues of citizenship and access to social rights of children, adolescents, youth, and adults in processes of ruptured social support networks (Barros, Ghirardi, & Lopes, 2002).

instability—often disrupt social participation and cohesion (Castel, 1998). Those affected experience daily discrimination, stigma, violence, and the violation of their rights, both through institutional systems and in everyday life.

Throughout my professional journey, I rooted my practice in social occupational therapy, using it as a technical foundation while drawing theoretical insight from education, sociology, anthropology, and philosophy. These disciplines provided a critical framework that enabled me to develop a thoughtful, engaged, and socially responsive approach.

What I am proposing here is not to evaluate specific models of practice or theoretical and methodological frameworks. Instead, through this autobiographical exploration, it is about seeking to identify elements for an occupational therapy praxis that departs from a biological and pragmatic interpretation of social reality. This embraces alternative theoretical perspectives to better understand the complexities and interconnections within the everyday lives and occupations of individuals and communities. This praxis moves beyond the traditional therapeutic setting, engaging with the spaces where daily life unfolds. It is ethically and politically committed, challenges hierarchical structures of power and knowledge, promotes respect for individual choices, and encourages critical reflection. Ultimately, it aims to enhance practice with both technical and scientific rigor (Lopes et al., 2014).

According to Silva et al. (2019), for the decolonization of knowledge and practices for occupational therapies, it is necessary to study "the processes of creation, production, and reproduction of these mechanisms of domination and exploitation" (p. 173) of people, groups, and communities historically marginalized by the processes of colonization. Thus, occupational therapists must begin to question the social and cultural gears that place individuals and groups in marginal places, producing and reproducing material arrangements, codes, and representations, in order to then think about intervention strategies in the field in which life takes place so that these transit between the macro- and the microsocial (Miskolci & Pelucio, 2011).

In the praxis of occupational therapy, it is essential to consider space not only from its physical but also its symbolic, cultural, and especially political dimensions, as these shape the mechanisms of coexistence in social life and influence daily activities and occupations. Spaces are often defined by restrictions and marginalization, creating places and non-places designated for certain bodies (Braga et al., 2020). Social markers such as race, gender, sexuality, and age play a crucial role in shaping ways of living and occupations for different groups, influencing destinies and shaping strategies of existence. Thus, occupational therapy must understand how individuals navigate the concrete conditions of their existence—and often survival—within the context of everyday life.

As a professor and researcher at a public university in Brazil, I have been developing work and research with young people and with the LGBTQIAP+ population, from an intersectional reading, betting on community and territorial work to approach, apprehend, and develop occupational therapy. I seek to contribute to creating creative strategies[13] to face the problems that cross the activities/occupations in conjunction with public policies. Even in the face of discourses, practices, and institutions that organize, reproduce, control, and standardize (Foucault, 1993), we have strategies of resistance, agency, and micropowers that go against hegemonic premises, creating new ways of *ser y estar*[14] to deconstruct and question the status quo.

These occupational therapy actions focus on creating strategies to strengthen social support networks and thinking from the micro- to the macrosocial level, and to favor the development of each subject's capacity for creation that allows them to appropriate reality, (re)create the world, and relate to others. Associated with this, it aims to build collective actions that have as a premise the identification and resolution of problems common to the subjects based on greater autonomy and social insertion from the assumptions of the exercise of democracy and the rights derived from citizenship (Lopes et al., 2014).

Thus, I have committed myself to the task of being a social articulator, creating qualified and ethical strategies in the outline of what it is to be an occupational therapist, producing together the opening to so many ways in which life can be produced, incorporating knowledge that meets the different social demands.

Interweaving categories: Deconstructing intersectionalities

We understand human beings as being and doing socially and culturally constituted in discursive wefts, in which gender, sexual orientation, class, ethnicity, belief, and generation are expressed, among other markers of difference. After sharing our autobiographical journeys, we identified that several categories dynamically intersect in these voices and gazes, as we develop below.

From the key of reading intersectionalities, we identify connections, confluences, and differentiations (Piscitelli, 2008), particularly in the category

13 I highlight the academic production by Alcântara et al. (2022) about artistic and urban interventions built with young people from a community to question and reflect on everyday life and the spaces used.

14 In Spanish, *ser* and *estar* both translate to "being" in English but convey different aspects of existence. *Ser* refers to an inherent, time-bound state of being (e.g., identity, essence, or permanence). In contrast *estar* refers to a situational, space-bound state of being (e.g., location, condition, or temporary states).

"women." We propose to look beyond the binary categorization, placing the experience of women in an ethical-political perspective, valuing the intersections between the various social markers of difference, which determine places of circulation and belonging, different experiences, and daily lives (Piscitelli, 2002).

We consider that being women and seeing ourselves (instead of being seen passively), talking about ourselves (instead of being judged), being subjective, and recognizing that what we have been, what we are, is also valuable, is a way of resisting homogenization and uprooting, typical of colonial and patriarchal thinking. We find in our narratives other possible forms of identification and praxis, exercising (or not) occupational therapy, giving place and voice to counter-hegemonic epistemologies and methodologies, which emerge from the desire to do, historicized and in otherness, in contrast to what should be.

In this context, Latin American women constantly move and transform at different historical, political, and cultural crossroads. A movement that represents transformations, displacements, changes, transfigurations, flows, and fluidity. We observe how narratives' ways of life—with their social, cultural, and political crossings, social participation, and praxis—shape, at the same time, unique narratives but also reverberate in collective processes in the construction of occupational therapies, in the plural.

Analyzing autobiographical stories allows us to give a decolonial perspective to praxis. It suggests that articulating the technical, ethical, and political dimensions of professional practice, moving between the individual and the collective, overcoming the theory–practice dichotomy, and constantly reaffirming the commitment to the transformation of society are essential dimensions for reflecting on professional practice. Situated in the dialectical relationship between society and history, this exercise of producing knowledge and doings around identities and praxis has allowed us to weave our networks of relationships, extending singular expressions to the collective (Cardinalli, 2017).

Reflecting on the collective, we find as an everyday accent the experience of the COVID-19 pandemic, in which the instrumentalization of death reminded us that we exercise a profession immersed in systems of ordering and social control, in which health is seen as a service, and in its less ethical expression, as a business in which being part of historically oppressed and marginalized groups limits the possibilities of living. This necropolitics[15]

15 "Necropolitics is the way of exercising sovereignty that is based on the expansion of colonial logic, since the reproduction of the objective and subjective conditions of economic life is established by the constant depreciation of material life, by the imprisonment of desire in the form of commodity and by the financialization of all spheres of life" (Almeida, 2021, p. 9).

(Mbembe, 2018) reflects governments' lack of effective action to mitigate these problems and ensure universal access to food, water, housing, and other fundamental social rights.

Another critical dimension of professional practice is the establishment of alliances and exchanges with other occupational therapists in the perspective of confronting the processes of precariousness and alienation of work, thinking about collective organization and mobilization in the face of models of institutional productivism, as well as strengthening a critical reading of work relations and processes (Bezerra, Lopes, & de Souza Basso, 2022).

To feel and think about occupational therapies requires a change in the way of understanding life and the everyday, outside of the colonizing and delimiting axes of creative possibility, prioritizing the realization of life with possibilities of autonomy and social participation. In Latin America, there is no way of producing professional practices without reflecting on the ways of life, the vulnerabilities, the differences and inequalities, mainly socio-economic, gender, sexuality, and race, and the daily lives of subjects and collectives.

These provocations are a liberating howl that strips us of the masks with which we hide other beings, knowledges, and doings that we also are that make us unique. We renounce the shame of fitting into groups, guilds, and homogenizing societies and free them from their bonds. They also encourage us to dialogue "face to face" with those voices that inhabit us, especially those that have been rejected or that we believe deserve our attention.

We weave these points of tension with careful and respectful ties, which locate other practices, voices, and possibilities for the construction of occupational therapy. Our experiences of migration and transit through territories in Latin America and Europe have made visible the tendency toward hegemonic practices of the profession where models such as the healthcare model, based mainly on Anglo-Saxon practices and protocols and laws that limit labor access under equal conditions, predominate.

Another point of reflection that connects us as women from the South is the production of care in occupational therapy based on decolonial axes and anchored in critical perspectives. We call for care practices that problematize standard and normative structures, models, and protocols, consider ancestry and local knowledge, value culture and individual and collective ways of life, and promote social participation and the radical exercise of democracy.

This cry for independence is also a call to self-knowledge to self-critically inhabit, occupy, live, leave the automatic pilot, and trace paths different from the determinisms that sustain the capitalist matrix, as Pérez (2021) mentioned. Abolishing any form of slavery and discrimination is today a challenge that depends on our everyday modes of re-production and consumption. We decide to let go of these devices of self-discipline (such as those we mentioned with self-censorship), and—taking up Professor Pérez (2021)—to move forward, identifying the imprints of the modern colonial matrix in order to move toward the construction of social knowledge from the South.

Conclusions

Reflecting collectively allowed us to recognize the emergence of generations of Latin American occupational therapists, whose identities and praxis were consolidated on the margins, in spaces of resistance and re-existence, due to realities marked by patriarchal and colonial traces and social injustice and violence. Confessing among peers, we rejoice that we have not mechanically reproduced a duty to be/do in each virtual meeting. However, instead, we venture into new experiences and form ourselves as researchers, broadening our horizons critically and proactively. Recalling private stories, we gave meaning to demand experiences, and we turned a voluntary space into an opportunity for personal and professional growth, to accompany us, to listen to and get to know us.

After deconstructing our stories in autobiographical accounts, we concluded that respect for and recognition of other ways of being and doing as individuals, families, guilds, societies, and humanity are imperative and that we must join forces toward decolonial, intersubjective, and intercultural approaches. As inhabitants of the same "big house," we can be agents of social transformation, vehicles, bridges, and channels of messages and actions that allow us to experience the joy of occupations. What do you say, do you join us?

References

Alcântara, A. C., Carvalho, C. D., Morais, H., Medeiros, N. M. S., et al. (2022). "Bem-vindo(a) ao meu timbó": Intervenções urbanas e arte pública com jovens de uma comunidade em João Pessoa. *Revista Interinstitucional Brasileira de Terapia Ocupacional, 6*(3), 1065–1074. https://doi.org/10.47222/2526-3544.rbto53309

Almeida, S. L. D. (2021). Necropolítica e neoliberalismo. *Caderno Crh, 34*, e021023. https://doi.org/10.9771/ccrh.v34i0.45397

Arendt, H. (2005). *The Human Condition* (R. Gil Novales, Transl.). Barcelona: Paidós.

Barros, D. D. D., Ghirardi, M. I. G., & Lopes, R. E. (2002). Social occupational therapy. *Revista Terapia Ocupacional da Universidade de São Paulo, 13*(3), 95–103. https://doi.org/10.11606/issn.2238-6149.v13i3p95-103

Becerra-Becerra, A. P. (2011). Caracolas itinerantes: Violence, occupational changes, and migrant women. In D. I. Munevar (Ed.), *De las Violencias Que Encierran a las Acciones Que Sanan*. Universidad Nacional de Colombia.

Becerra-Becerra, A. P., & Moreno-Sosa, M. (2003). Occupational therapy perspectives on HIV/AIDS: An experience of VIHDA. *Revista Ocupación Humana, 10*(1–2), 27–39. https://doi.org/10.25214/25907816.660

Bezerra, W. C., Lopes, R. E., & de Souza Basso, A. C. (2022). As estruturas da vida cotidiana e a terapia ocupacional: Tensionando limites e possibilidades no/do exercício profissional. *Cadernos Brasileiros De Terapia Ocupacional, 30*, e3031. https://doi.org/10.1590/2526-8910.ctoEN22983031

Birulés, F. (2015). *Entreactos. En Torno a la Política, el Feminismo y el Pensamiento*. Madrid: Katz Editores.

Bondía, J. L. (2002). Notes on experience and the knowledge of experience. *Revista Brasiliera Educação, 19*. https://doi.org/10.1590/S1413-24782002000100003

Braga, I. F., Melo, K. M. M. M., Monzeli, G. A., Leite Junior, J. D., Farias, M. N., & Correia, R. L. (2020). Crise da democracia brasileira e o cotidiano de pessoas dissidentes de gêneros e sexualidades: Reflexões baseadas na terapia ocupacional social. *Cadernos Brasileiros de Terapia Ocupacional, 28*(2), 693–705. https://doi.org/10.4322/2526-8910.ctoARF1958

Brazilian Government. Decree 6.040 of 07 February 2007. www.planalto.gov.br/ccivil_03/_ato2007-2010/2007/decreto/d6040.htm

Butler, J. (2004). *Language, Power, and Identity*. Madrid: Síntesis.

Butler, J. (2006). *Gender Trouble: Feminism and the Subversion of Identity*. London: Routledge.

Cantero Garlito, P. A., Émeric Méaule, D., Zango Martín, I., & Domínguez Vega, E. (2012). Women's occupations, men's occupations: The influence of gender on occupation and the occupational therapy profession in Spain. *TOG (A Coruña), 9*(5), 96–124. www.revistatog.com/mono/num5/genero.pdf

Cardinalli, I. (2017). *Conhecimentos da terapia ocupacional no Brasil: Um estudo sobre trajetórias e produções*. Dissertation. São Carlos: UFSCar.

Castel, R. (1998). *As Metamorfoses da Questão Social: Uma Crônica do Salário* (I. D. Poleti, Trans.). Vozes.

Castillo Aguas, J. P., & Varón Caicedo, V. (2017). Desempeño ocupacional realizante: Una mirada a su trayectoria, aportes a su fundamentación teórica. *Revista Ocupación Humana, 17*(1), 7–24. https://latinjournal.org/index.php/roh/article/view/153

de Figueiredo, A. V. (2011). *O Caminho Quilombola: Sociologia Jurídica do Reconhecimento Étnico*. Editora Appris.

Foucault, M. (1993). *Microfísica do Poder*. Rio de Janeiro: Edições Graal.

Freire, P. (1970). The adult literacy process as cultural action for freedom. *Harvard Educational Review, 40*(2), 205–225.

Freire de Araújo Lima, E. M., & Lima de Paula, I. (2023). Mujeres, feminismo y terapia ocupacional: Un análisis crítico de la literatura sobre las cuestiones de género que afectan a la profesión. *Revista Ocupación Humana, 23*(2). https://doi.org/10.25214/25907816.1583

Galheigo, S. M. (2012). Perspectiva crítica y compleja de terapia ocupacional: Actividad, cotidiano, diversidad, justice social y compromisso ético-político. *TOG (A Coruña), 9*(5), 176–197.

Galheigo, S. M., Braga, C. P., Arthur, M. A., & Matsuo, C. M. (2018). Produção de conhecimento, perspectivas e referências teórico-práticas na terapia ocupacional brasileira: Marcos e tendências em uma linha do tempo. *Cadernos Brasileiros De Terapia Ocupacional, 26*(4), 723–738. https://doi.org/10.4322/2526-8910.ctoAO1773

García-Ruiz, S. (2016). Occupational therapy in Colombia. In S. Simó, A. Guajardo, O. F. Correa, S. M. Galheigo, & S. García (Eds.), *Terapias Ocupacionales desde el Sur: Derechos Humanos, Ciudadanía y Participación* (pp. 81–84). Universidad Santiago de Chile.

Lejeune, P. (1991). The autobiographical pact: Autobiography and its theoretical problems. *Anthropos Supplements*, (29), 47–61.

Lopes, R. E., Malfitano, A. P. S., Silva, C. R., & Borba, P. L. (2014). Recursos e tecnologias em terapia ocupacional social: Ações com jovens pobres na cidade. *Cadernos de Terapia Ocupacional da UFSCar, 22*(3), 591–602. https://doi.org/10.4322/cto.2014.081

López, Y. (2019). *Sociopoética y différance de la ocupación en la (de)construcción auto-biográfica de docentes colombianos y españoles*. Doctoral thesis, University of Zaragoza. https://zaguan.unizar.es/record/78880

López Díaz, Y. P. (2015). La autobiografía (de)constructura del que-hacer-se educativo. *Tropelías: Revista De Teoría De La Literatura Y Literatura Comparada*, no. 23, 73–89. https://dialnet.unirioja.es/servlet/articulo?codigo=4931948

Malfitano, A. P. S. (2016). Contexto social e atuação social: Generalizações e especificidades na terapia ocupacional. In R. E. Lopes & A. P. S. Malfitano (Eds.), *Terapia Ocupacional Social: Desenhos Teóricos e Contornos Práticos* (pp. 117–134). São Carlos: EDUFSCar.

Mbembe, A. (2018). *Necropolitics: Biopower, Sovereignty, State of Exclusion, Politics of Death*. São Paulo: N-1 Edições.

Miskolci, R., & Pelucio, L. (2011). *Discursos Fora da Ordem: Sexualidades, Saberes e Direitos*. São Paulo: Annablume; Fapesp.

Mora Augier, C. (2022). Mujeres, aberes y profesiones: Un recorrido desde las ciencias sociales de Ana Laura Martin, Graciela Queirolo y Karina Ramacciotti (coords.) (2019) Editorial Biblos, 204 pp. *Estudios Sociales Del Estado, 8*(15). https://doi.org/10.35305/ese.v8i15.293

Núñez, C. M. V. (2019). Terapias ocupacionales del Sur: Una propuesta para su comprensión. *Cadernos Brasileiros de Terapia Ocupacional, 27*(3), 671–680.

Pérez, L. (2021). *Ocupación Humana: De la Matriz Colonial Moderna hacia la Construcción de Saberes Sociales del Sur*. Bogotá: Universidad Nacional de Colombia. Facultad de Medicina. Centro editorial.

Piscitelli, A. (2002). Recriando a (categoria) mulher? In L. M. Algranti (Org.), *A Prática Feminista e o Conceito de Gênero. Textos Didáticos*. Campinas, IFCH.

Piscitelli, A. (2008). Intersectionalidades, categorias de articulação e experiências de migrantes brasileiras. *Sociedade e Cultura, 11*(2), 263–274. https://doi.org/10.5216/sec.v11i2.5247

Reiter, B. (2016). Los Wintukua: Los guardianos del mundo. *Memorias: Revista Digital de Historia y Arqueologia desde el Caribe*, (28), 1–28.

Rodó-Zárate, M. (2021). *Intersectionality. Inequalities, Places, and Emotions*. Bellaterra Edicions, Manresa.

Silva, C. R., Jarra, R. M., Calle del Campo, Y., & Kronenberg, F. (2019). Terapias ocupacionais do Sul: Demandas atuais a partir de uma perspectiva socio-histórica. *Revisbrato, 3*(2), 172–178. https://doi.org/10.47222/2526-3544.rbto24867

Silvestrini, M. S., Silva, C. R., & Prado, A. C. D. S. A. (2019). Occupational therapy and culture: Ethical-political dimensions and resistances. *Cadernos Brasileiros de Terapia Ocupacional, 27*, 929–940.

Simó, S. (2016). Terapia ocupacional, cultura y diversidad. *Cadernos de Terapia Ocupacional da UFSCar, 24*(1), 163–171. http://dx.doi.org/10.4322/0104-4931.ctoRE0677

Sória, S. (2023). Academic practice and intersectionality: Notes from Latin American postcoloniality. *Debate Feminista, 66*, 1–28. https://doi.org/10.22201/cieg.2594066xe.2023.66.2361

Turcotte, P. L., & Holmes, D. (2021). The (dis)obedient occupational therapist: A reflection on dissent against disciplinary propaganda. *Cadernos Brasileiros de Terapia Ocupacional, 29*, e2924. https://doi.org/10.1590/2526-8910.ctoARF2211

UNESCO (2023). Ancestral system of knowledge of the four indigenous peoples, Arhuaco, Kankuamo, Kogui and Wiwa of the Sierra Nevada de Santa Marta. https://ich.unesco.org/en/RL/ancestral-system-of-knowledge-of-the-four-indigenous-peoples-arhuaco-kankuamo-kogui-and-wiwa-of-the-sierra-nevada-de-santa-marta-01886

CHAPTER 5

Exploring the Roots of the Southern Occupational Therapies

A MOSAIC OF PRACTICES AND PERSPECTIVES

Livet Rocío Cristancho, María Cristina Fernández Orellana, Sara M. Daneri, and Elizabeth Rodríguez Uzcátegui

With contributions from: Alicia Herrera Bonilla, Gabriela Elizabeth Navarrete Rodríguez, Andrés Rey, Andrea F. Albino, Orlando Enrique Pérez, María Pedernera, and Ecuador's and Paraguay's CLATO Delegates

Abstract

This chapter delves into the origins and evolution of occupational therapies in Latin America, highlighting key milestones and the unique development of the profession across the region. It examines professional identity construction within local contexts, focusing on the influence of Global North paradigms and the emergence of Southern perspectives. The chapter traces the historical development of occupational therapy from 1840 to 1950, emphasizing factors such as moral treatment approaches, responses to epidemics, and international collaborations. It also details the expansion of education and practice from 1971 to 2022, noting the establishment of new programs and the impact of sociopolitical changes, including neoliberal policies and community-based approaches. The role of professional associations in shaping the profession is discussed, alongside the impact of global and local political contexts on training programs. The chapter critically examines the profession's trajectory through a collaborative methodology involving occupational therapists from various countries, reflecting on colonial influences, social and political contexts, and emerging identities distinct from Global North models. It provides a comprehensive overview of the profession's evolution in Latin America, addressing contemporary challenges and future directions.

Keywords
occupational therapy; Latin America; occupational therapies of the South; professional identity; origins of occupational therapy

Learning outcomes

- Analyze the historical and epistemological foundations of occupational therapy in Latin America, considering how local customs, beliefs, and practices influenced the profession's development in the region.
- Discuss the evolution of occupational therapy practices in Latin America, examining how professional identity transformed in response to regional and local contexts and how this relates to current research and significant areas of practice.
- Critically examine the influence of global political and economic factors on the development of occupational therapy education and practice in Latin America.
- Discuss the role of professional associations and international collaborations in shaping the identity and growth of occupational therapy in the region.

Introduction

This chapter delves into the development of occupational therapy in Latin America from a distinctly Southern perspective, aiming to trace key milestones that shaped the profession and its identity across the region. The authors, all of whom have been actively engaged in national and regional professional organizations like the Latin American Confederation of Occupational Therapy (CLATO),[1] provide their perspective on how occupational therapy emerged in Latin America, shaped by the region's unique historical, sociopolitical, and cultural landscapes.

We begin by addressing the geographical and conceptual definitions of

1 CLATO (in Spanish, Confederación Latinoamericana de Terapeutas Ocupacionales) is a regional organization representing occupational therapists in Latin America. It was founded in 1997 in Venezuela during the 3rd Latin American Congress on Occupational Therapy. As of 2019, its member countries included Argentina, Bolivia, Brazil, Chile, Colombia, Costa Rica, El Salvador, Mexico, Panama, Paraguay, Peru, Puerto Rico, Uruguay, and Venezuela. CLATO aims to develop the occupational therapy profession in the Latin American region, strengthen professional identity, and expand fields of practice and international cooperation between associations, institutions, and organizations in member countries. It also organizes Latin American Congresses of Occupational Therapy every two years to facilitate knowledge exchange.

Latin America, recognizing that it is not simply a region defined by borders but one deeply influenced by historical and sociopolitical factors, particularly the oppressions of the Global North. Aráujo (2006) and Souza (2012) noted that Latin America comprises 32 countries south of the Rio Grande in Mexico. However, some definitions limit the region to 20 Spanish, Portuguese, and French-speaking nations. Regardless of the definition, it is essential to acknowledge the profound historical forces of colonialism and Northern oppressions that influenced the region's population, economy, and cultural identity.

The chapter explores how the global division between the "north" and "south," as metaphorically represented by de Sousa Santos (2018), influenced the construction of occupational therapy in Latin America. The profession initially adopted Eurocentric knowledge and practices, primarily influenced by the United States and Europe, often incongruent with local cultural and social contexts. Over time, however, Southern occupational therapies emerged, focusing on integrating local narratives, cultural transformations, and regional knowledge, as Valderrama (2019) and Díaz and Malfitano (2021) emphasized.

We examine the profession's emergence across countries like Argentina, Chile, Colombia, Ecuador, Panama, Paraguay, Peru, Uruguay, and Venezuela, analyzing how diverse national contexts influenced its development. Notably, we distinguish between the discipline of occupational therapy—its theoretical frameworks and concepts—and the profession, which encompasses the practical application of this knowledge in various sectors. Universities played a crucial role in shaping the discipline and the profession,[2] creating scientific foundations that continue to inform practice (Ayala, 2019).

The chapter is structured around four major milestones in the development of occupational therapy in the region:

- The First Milestone: Initial steps into the profession and key factors shaping the emergence of occupational therapy (1840–1950).
- The Second Milestone: Advancing the profession in the region, new programs, and developments in occupational therapy (1971–1995).
- The Third Milestone: The expansion of occupational therapy training

2 In this chapter, we differentiate between discipline and profession within the context of occupational therapy. The discipline refers to the theoretical foundations, concepts, and frameworks that constitute the body of knowledge in the field. It is shaped by academic institutions, which develop and refine these ideas. On the other hand, the profession encompasses the practical application of this knowledge, focusing on the work performed by occupational therapists in various sectors. Universities play a key role in advancing the discipline, while practitioners apply these scientific foundations in their profession.

in Latin America (1996–2022) and the impact of the COVID-19 pandemic.
- The Fourth Milestone: Professional associations as a dynamic and integrative force for occupational therapy in Southern countries.

Through collaborative research and historical accounts, the narrative provides a nuanced understanding of how occupational therapy evolved in this region, addressing its practitioners' unique challenges.

Our goal is to contribute to a broader understanding of the profession's development by weaving together historical, political, economic, and cultural influences, creating a rich context for analyzing how Latin American occupational therapists have constructed their professional identity amid the distinct challenges of the Global South.

The First Milestone: Initial steps into the profession and key factors shaping the emergence of occupational therapy (1840–1950)

The role of moral treatment, labor therapy, and activity-based interventions

Occupational therapy's roots in Latin America can be traced to the late 18th and 19th centuries, when practices were developed to address physical and mental well-being through structured occupation and labor. These early practices served therapeutic goals while addressing broader social issues, such as managing marginalized populations and preventing vagrancy. These practices were adapted according to local needs and cultural contexts.

During colonial times, hospitals were established in the region to address social-health challenges, often from a philanthropic perspective (Duarte et al., 2016). "Labor therapy" (or "ergotherapy") was one of the key therapeutic tools used to rehabilitate individuals with mental health issues. This practice focused on tailoring activities to individuals' needs, aligning with historical references to "Types of Madness" (MacDonald, 1972). Moral treatment was central to mental health care in Europe and North America, emphasizing structured activities and work to restore mental well-being (Trujillo, 1989).

Table 5.1 provides an overview of how various Latin American countries applied these early occupational therapy principles, including Colombia's use of work and trades in asylums and Venezuela's labor therapy programs in psychiatric hospitals. The scope of application, target populations, and specific occupational methods varied across the region but shared the common goal of rehabilitation and social reintegration.

Table 5.1 Occupational therapy's use of activities and occupations to address health issues

Country	Reference names of the profession	Resource used	Scope of application	Target	Function
Colombia (Duarte et al., 2016; Garcia et al., 2022; Trujillo, 1989, 2002)	Use of work and occupations; labor therapy, play therapy, or ergotherapy.	Use of work and trades since the 17th century.	Linked to charity and philanthropy in asylums, hospices, and sanatoriums in Medellín, Bucaramanga, and Bogotá.	Re-educate habits and train or educate for work. Linked to charity and philanthropy. To create manpower for production in the country's companies and to attend to health problems.	Empirical way of dealing with mental health problems; a response to issues of marginality and social disorder; a means of dealing with sensory impairment or mental retardation.
Venezuela (de Oliveira, 2000)	Laboratory therapy.	Workshops for baking, pottery, sewing, agriculture, and animal husbandry.	Psychiatric hospitals.	Respond to the immediate needs of asylum seekers and provide savings in case of discharge. Generate resources for the state.	The production fed the towns of Catia and Sucre as well as hospitals.
Argentina (Botinelli et al., 2016; Daneri, 2005)	Laboratory therapy.	Printing workshop, broom making, carpentry, rural work.	Asylums, hospices, psychiatric colonies, psychiatric hospitals.	Use of labor as a method of discipline. Restore moral order. Generate resources for the state and be self-sustainable.	Isolation and asylum to address mental health issues and contain social disorder.
Paraguay (Oral story by occupational therapist Ingrid Aquino)	Laboratory therapy.	Vegetable garden workshop, literary workshop, hairdressing services, donation of used clothes, fruit, carpentry, handicraft, sports and recreational activities.	Psychiatric hospitals.	Mennonite Voluntary Service (SERVOME).	Responding to the shortcomings of the care system and the lack of activity and occupation.
Ecuador (Stucchi, 2015)	Use of work.	Manual labor and agricultural production.	Psychiatric hospitals.	Stimulating and regularizing organic functions and a powerful moral agent.	Economic self-sufficiency.

As can be seen, occupation-based therapies played a significant role in managing mental health and social challenges in several Latin American countries. In Colombia, labor therapy was linked to charitable efforts in asylums and focused on preparing individuals for work. Similarly, in Venezuela and Argentina, labor therapy in psychiatric hospitals aimed to restore moral order and generate resources for the state.

These practices reflected broader social and economic goals, with occupations such as baking, carpentry, and agricultural work used to manage mental health issues and social order. In Paraguay and Ecuador, labor therapy programs were tailored to the specific needs of psychiatric patients, focusing on skills development and economic self-sufficiency. This adaptive approach to occupational therapy is summarized in Table 5.1.

Technical collaboration and international partnerships: The impact of the polio epidemic and regional vulnerability

The development of occupational therapy in Latin America was heavily influenced by the social and health challenges posed by the polio epidemic in the mid-20th century. As Table 5.2 illustrates, international partnerships played a critical role in responding to the epidemic, leading to the establishment of occupational therapy programs in countries such as Argentina, Chile, and Venezuela.

The polio epidemic primarily affected children, highlighted the lack of local human resources, and prompted collaboration with foreign professionals. Volunteers and students were among the first to receive occupational therapy training, often through international cooperation agreements. These collaborations involved organizations like the World Health Organization (WHO), Pan American Health Organization (PAHO), and International Labor Organization (ILO), as outlined in Table 5.2.

During this period, international cooperation facilitated the establishment of rehabilitation services across the region. For example, in Venezuela and Argentina, occupational therapy programs were launched in 1959, marking the beginning of formal occupational therapy education in Latin America. These programs laid the foundation for similar initiatives in other countries, including Chile, Colombia, and Peru. The box following Table 5.2 provides additional examples of how international cooperation contributed to developing the first occupational therapy programs in the region. The partnerships between foreign experts and local institutions were essential in addressing the polio epidemic and advancing the profession in Latin America.

Table 5.2 Country responses to the polio epidemic and social factors: Actions and international cooperation

Country	Country response to polio cases; other factors, social and labor	Actions carried out	International cooperation agency	Cooperative actions in response to the epidemic and social and employment factors
Venezuela (Monzeli, 2019; Rivas et al., 2013)	1936–1937 People with mental disabilities.	Employment of European staff at the Psychiatric Hospital of Caracas. Employment of an American occupational therapist specializing in mental health and neuromotor rehabilitation.		Care for people with mental disorders.
	1944 Accidents at work and occupational diseases.	Creation of the Venezuelan Social Security Institute (IVSS).		Scholarships for training in industrial medicine.
	1954	IVSS pilot Rehabilitation Centre for the Disabled, La Guaira.	UN	Auxiliary training.
Argentina (Albino, 2022; Botinelli et al., 2016; Nabergoi, 2013; Testa, 2012, 2013)	1956 A major epidemic that prompted the Argentine government to negotiate international agreements for the care of the thousands of children affected by polio.	Creation of the National Commission for Cripple Rehabilitation (CNRL) and management of foreign professionals.	WHO PAHO ILO National government and the British Council	
	1957			Occupational therapy assistant training courses by Elizabeth Hollings and Ruby Kroom.

Chile (Monzeli, 2019)	1947 Creation at the private level of the Asociación Pro-Ayuda al Niño Lisiado, now called Instituto Teletón.		PAHO ILO	
	1952	Enactment of the National Health Service Law n°10.383 allocated funds for rehabilitation.		
	1957	Creation of the Pedro Aguirre Cerda Children's Rehabilitation Centre.	Hellen Wessel and Kellogg Foundations (1959)	In 1959, a doctor traveled to the US on a scholarship for training in physiatry.
Colombia (Duarte et al., 2016; Trujillo, 2002)	1959 Establishment of the Franklin D. Roosevelt Institute for rehabilitating children with orthopedic and neuromuscular problems. The first occupational therapy service for physical dysfunction was started at the San Juan de Dios Hospital in Bogotá.		An occupational therapist from the United States	Creation of the occupational therapy service.

Examples of How International Cooperation Led to the First Occupational Therapy Programs in Latin America

Venezuela

In 1959, the National School of Rehabilitation, now known as the May Hamilton University College of Rehabilitation, was established. This institution was set up to provide a dual qualification as a physiotherapist and occupational therapist, which later was separated into two distinct programs, following the World Federation of Occupational Therapy and the World Federation of Physiotherapy recommendations, which advocated separate course designs. The initiative was supported by international experts, including occupational therapist May Hamilton and physiotherapist Katherine de Brecht from the United Nations, alongside the Universidad Central de Venezuela. This collaboration laid the foundation for professional training in rehabilitation in the country (Rivas et al., 2013).

Further advancements in occupational therapy education took place in 1967 when the Faculty of Medicine, School of Public Health, launched the first Occupational Therapy Course through an agreement between PAHO, WHO, the Ministry of Health and Social Development, and the Universidad Central de Venezuela. This initiative aimed to establish regional rehabilitation services, particularly for individuals with leprosy, a significant public health concern at the time. An international consultant, Argentine occupational therapist Carmen Forn de Zita, was hired to develop and lead the program (Rivas et al., 2013).

Argentina

1959 marked the creation of Argentina's first National School of Occupational Therapy. This effort was spearheaded by English occupational therapist Evelyn Mary Macdonald and her team of colleagues from England. Their contribution was pivotal in establishing formal education and training for occupational therapists in Argentina, setting a precedent for the profession in the region (Bottinelli et al., 2016; Testa, 2012).

Chile

In 1961, a doctor trained as a psychiatrist in the United States returned to Chile and contributed to developing an occupational therapy proposal for rehabilitation treatment. The first Chilean occupational therapist was trained in Argentina, highlighting the regional cooperation in professional development. This regional cooperation involved sharing knowledge, resources, and best practice among countries in the region, which was crucial in the early stages of occupational therapy development. The National Health Service and the Pan American Health Organization (PAHO) coordinated efforts to strengthen services and train professionals. By 1963, Chile had launched its first experimental occupational therapy program at the University of Chile, linked to the School of Medical Technology. This program was officially constituted with the help of WHO consultant Margarita León de Pérez, who was trained in the USA (Guajardo, 2016; Monzeli et al., 2021; Morrison et al., 2016).

Colombia

The demand for rehabilitation services grew in 1964 due to violence, political confrontation, and social crises. This demand led to the involvement of American and Colombian occupational therapists, including Alicia Trujillo, a United States graduate. By 1966, technical academic programs in physical therapy, speech therapy, and occupational therapy were established, with contributions from graduates of the National University and those trained in Argentina. The Universidad del Rosario and the Colombian School of Rehabilitation began offering technical curricula, expanding professional practice areas to include physical and psychosocial dysfunctions. By 1969, these programs were affiliated with the Colombian Institute for the Promotion of Higher Education (ICFES), which standardized essential training criteria (Duarte et al., 2016; Trujillo, 2002, 2013).

Peru

The National Rehabilitation Institute was inaugurated in 1962 in the San Miguel district. Two Peruvian teachers were sent to study occupational therapy at the Mexican Institute of Rehabilitation, supported by a US Embassy scholarship. The School of Medical Technology was created at the Universidad Nacional Mayor de San Marcos (UNMSM) in 1966, beginning operations in 1967. By 1969, an academic program in occupational therapy was established at the Escuela Académico Profesional de Tecnología Médica at UNMSM, with the first cohort graduating in 1972 (Flores et al., 2021).

Global and local political contexts influencing the origin of occupational therapy training programs

The first occupational therapy academic programs in Latin America emerged within a context defined by social inequalities, healthcare accessibility challenges, and significant sociopolitical tensions that shaped public policies. According to Guajardo (2016), political efforts to address pressing social needs largely drove the establishment and consolidation of the occupational therapy profession. In countries such as Venezuela, Argentina, Peru, Chile, and Colombia, these developments often occurred under political regimes marked by dictatorship or intense ideological conflicts, which directly shaped the trajectory of occupational therapy programs, as detailed in the box below.

Examples of How Global and Local Political Contexts Influenced the Origin of Occupational Therapy Training Programs in Latin America

Venezuela

Before the establishment of its first occupational therapy training program in 1959, Venezuela was under a military dictatorship, which saw the creation of rehabilitation centers to address pressing health needs. However, even after the country transitioned to a constitutional government in 1959, it faced internal instability, including brief military rebellions and the rise of guerrilla movements influenced by the Cuban Revolution (Orovitz, 2009).

Argentina

In 1955, Argentina's political landscape shifted when a de facto government took power. In response to a major polio epidemic in 1956, the National Commission for the Rehabilitation of the Crippled was established, hiring English therapists to treat affected children. The first occupational therapy program was introduced in 1959 under a developmental constitutional government supported by international collaboration. However, the country experienced further political turmoil, including coups d'état, between 1962 and 1966 (Orovitz, 2009).

Chile

In the 1960s, Chile experienced sociopolitical transformations marked by debates between development and socialist models. The first occupational therapy program was established in 1963 during economic and social reforms aligned with United States policies (Biblioteca del Congreso Nacional de Chile, 2023; Escobar & Sepúlveda, 2013; Guajardo, 2016; Monzeli, 2019).

Colombia

Between 1960 and 1980, Colombia faced ongoing political strife between liberal and conservative parties, compounded by severe social issues, such as unemployment, poverty, and the aftermath of the polio epidemic. When the first occupational therapy program was launched in 1966, the country faced a political crisis, with guerrilla groups rising in response to social exclusion and unequal land distribution. Social reforms during this time, including the increased participation of women in higher education, also shaped the occupational therapy profession (Duarte et al., 2016; Rodríguez et al., 2016; Trujillo, 1989).

International cooperation was a significant factor in developing occupational therapy training programs before formalized local educational structures were in place. This collaboration took multiple forms: foreign professionals specializing in rehabilitation contributed expertise, returning scholars who had studied abroad brought back essential knowledge, and institutions dedicated to the care and rehabilitation of individuals affected by conditions like poliomyelitis, social violence, and occupational injuries were established. Despite the support, many countries faced an acute shortage of qualified healthcare personnel, which became a matter of public policy in countries like Argentina, Chile, Colombia, and Venezuela.

The sociopolitical landscape also contributed to these developments. For example, the Cuban Revolution spurred regional political and economic stability concerns, prompting the United States to launch the Alliance for Progress (1961–1970). This program provided economic, political, and social aid to Latin American countries aligned with US objectives. Through aid agencies, multilateral financial institutions, and private-sector partnerships, the United States contributed resources to improve social and health conditions across the region (Ramos & Castro, 2014). This influx of foreign theories, methods, and techniques often did not align with local cultural contexts, influencing the construction of the early professional identity of occupational therapists in Latin America.

Reflect and Discuss

- What is the background of occupational therapy in your region?
- What common characteristics do you identify with your country?
- What factors influenced the arrival of occupational therapy in the region?

- Can you identify cooperation from national or international organizations in creating your academic program? What were the reasons for the support received?
- Are there political, social, or economic factors among the countries in your region that have driven the creation of occupational therapy programs? If so, which ones?
- Are there any historical aspects that have influenced the creation of occupational therapy programs in your region, country, or city?

Second Milestone: Advancing the profession in the region, new programs, and developments in occupational therapy (1971–1995)

During the 1970s and 1980s, the development of the occupational therapy profession gained momentum across Latin America, marked by the establishment of new academic programs. In Ecuador, initial programs were launched in the late 1970s, and by the 1980s, foreign-trained professors were contributing specialized knowledge to the field (CLATO, n.d.). Bachelor's degree programs in Peru were developed within the *Licenciatura en Tecnología Médica* framework, specializing in occupational therapy (Flores et al., 2021).

The expansion of occupational therapy interventions continued in other countries during this period, although formal training programs were not always available. In Panama and Paraguay, foreign professionals played a significant role in providing services and supporting the profession's growth. In Uruguay, the political climate created unique challenges for establishing consistent academic training. Figure 5.1 provides an overview of these developments, highlighting various educational initiatives such as the launch of new programs and the revision of curricula and service initiatives like the initiation of new state programs in Panama, Ecuador, Paraguay, and Uruguay between 1965 and 1990.

Global and local political contexts influencing the development of occupational therapy in countries with previously established training programs

As shown in Figure 5.2, the development of occupational therapy in countries with established training programs faced challenges to progress during the 1970s and 1980s. In Argentina, several new programs were launched, but political upheavals, including military dictatorships, led to the closure of many. Similar disruptions occurred in Peru and Uruguay, where political instability hindered the continuity and establishment of training programs (Flores et al., 2021; Martínez, 2020; Sosa, 2019).

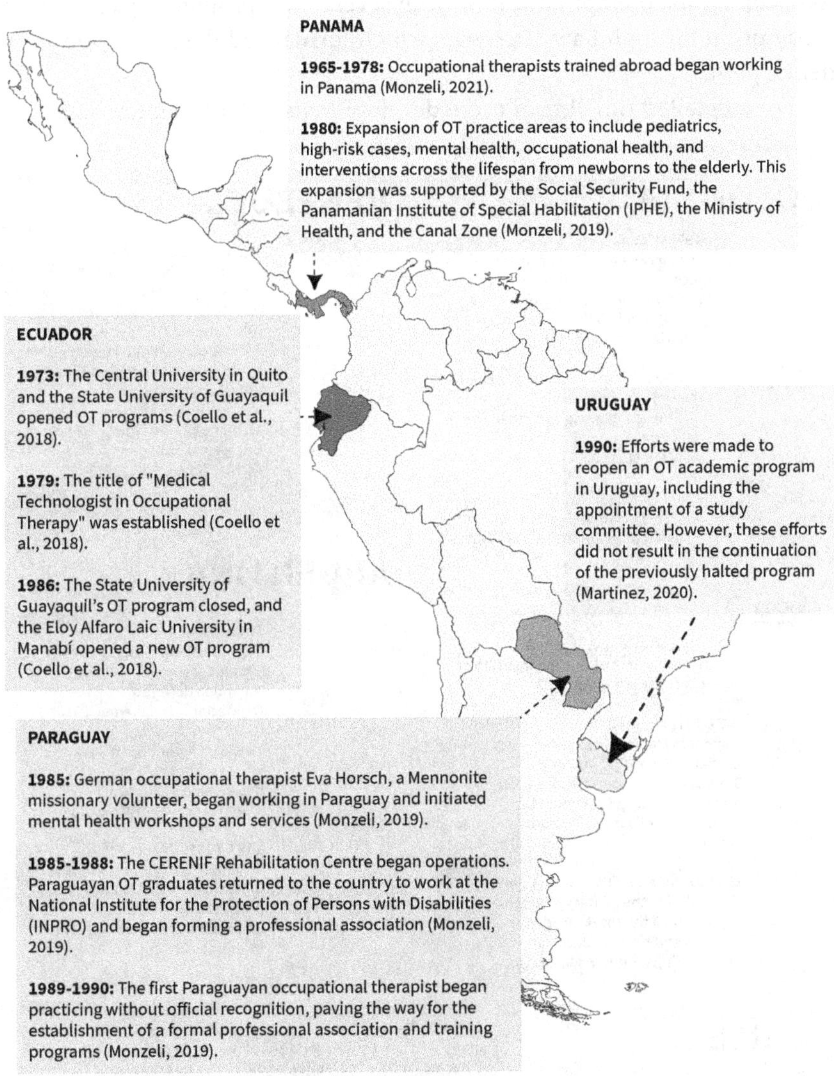

Figure 5.1 Examples of the development of occupational therapy training programs between 1965 and 1990 in Latin American countries (made by Pamela Talero)

This period was characterized by the repression of community-based mental health initiatives and professionals, particularly in Argentina and Chile, due to the sociopolitical climates of their respective dictatorships (Escobar &

Sepúlveda, 2013; Nabergoi, 2013). Despite these challenges, advancements were made. Countries like Chile revised their curricula to meet international standards, and Venezuela initiated new state programs. Colombia expanded its occupational therapy education with several new programs, gaining legal recognition through Law 100/1993, which formalized the profession's academic path.

For a detailed timeline of these developments, refer to Figure 5.2.

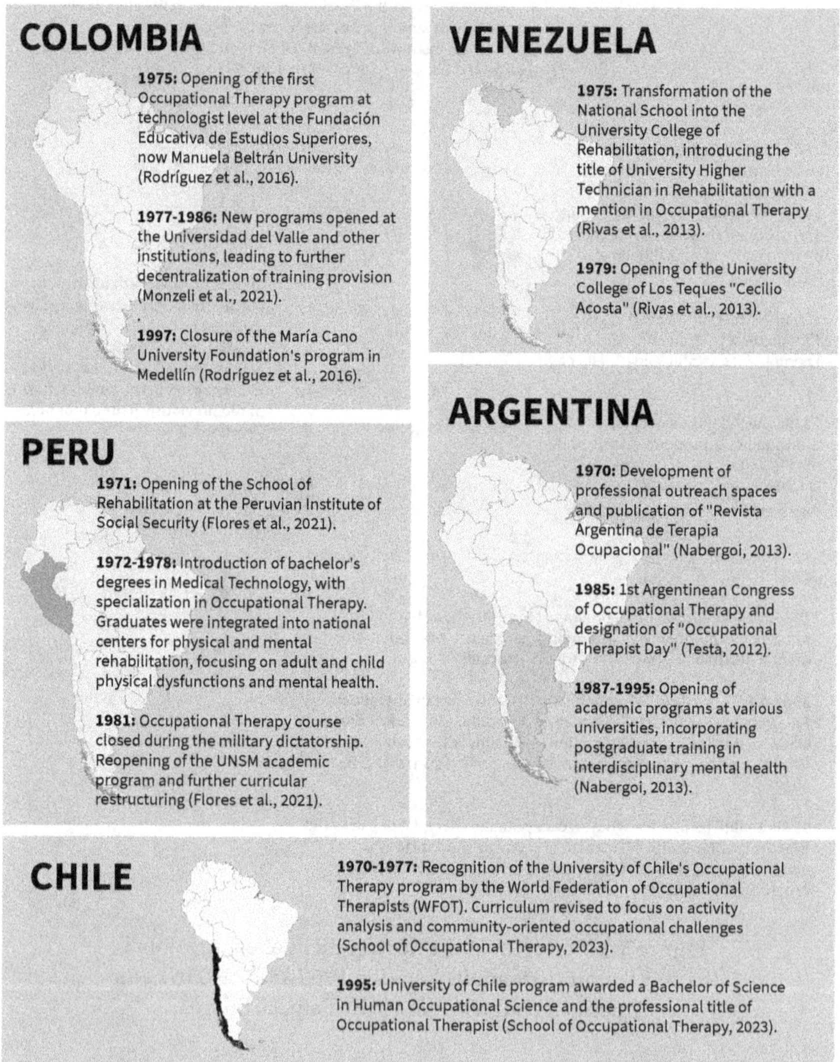

Figure 5.2 Continuity of occupational therapy development in selected Latin American countries (made by Pamela Talero)

Throughout the 1970s and 1980s, Latin America underwent profound political and social transformations that significantly influenced the development of occupational therapy in countries with established training programs. During the Cold War era, Soviet–Latin American relations were shaped by geopolitical tensions and ideological conflicts, as the Soviet Union sought to expand its influence in the region while the United States aimed to maintain control. This dynamic contributed to significant events such as coups d'état, the rise of military regimes, and the implementation of neoliberal policies that reshaped economic and social landscapes, particularly in the health and education sectors (Grandin, 2004). In response to perceived Soviet threats, the USA supported military coups and authoritarian regimes, with notable examples including the 1954 coup in Uruguay and Pinochet's 1973 coup in Chile (Blasier, 1987). These interventions, however, often targeted guerrilla movements that had emerged in response to systemic inequalities favoring US-backed elites, exacerbating regional instability. Many countries experienced substantial guerrilla movements and military conflicts, further complicating efforts to advance social sectors like health and education (Cristancho & Llanos, 2019; Katz, 2015; Rodríguez et al., 2016). As the Cold War ended, new trends in Soviet–Latin American relations emerged, reflecting the shifting political landscape in both regions (Mujal-León, 1989). While this summary highlights key events, the complexity of this era demands a more nuanced analysis to fully understand its lasting impact on professional fields like occupational therapy.

Neoliberal reforms, characterized by market liberalization and privatization, brought substantial changes to health and education. These reforms aligned with global initiatives such as the Alma-Ata Declaration (1978) and the Ottawa Charter (1986), which emphasized community participation and access to primary healthcare (Cristancho, 2021; Laurell, 2012). These shifts encouraged an expansion from clinical settings to community-based and social practices, reshaping occupational therapy's professional identity to focus on social inclusion, human rights, and broader social needs (Corrêa & Nicacio, 1999).

By the 1980s and 1990s, occupational therapy education evolved from technical training to more comprehensive professional programs driven by political and social crises that underscored the need for community-oriented practice. Reforms in countries like Argentina, Colombia, and Chile facilitated discussions on managing mental health and disability, emphasizing citizenship and participation (Orovitz, 2009).

During this period, occupational therapy practice expanded beyond traditional biomedical approaches to address poverty, substance abuse prevention, and social integration. This evolution was further shaped by local sociopolitical dynamics, natural disasters, and ongoing social challenges, leading to a diverse and inclusive approach to occupational therapy across the region (Monzeli et al., 2021; Rodriguez et al., 2016). Overall, these decades were pivotal in transitioning occupational therapy in Latin America from a predominantly clinical focus to a more community-centered approach, better aligned with broader social determinants of health and the unique sociopolitical landscape of the region.

The Third Milestone: The expansion of occupational therapy training in Latin America (1996–2022) and the impact of the COVID-19 pandemic

Between 1996 and 2022, occupational therapy education in Latin America experienced significant growth, marked by establishing new training programs across various countries. This expansion has greatly contributed to the professional development of occupational therapy in the region (Bianchi & Malfitano, 2017).

In Colombia, occupational therapy programs increased to 12, comprising nine private and three public institutions spread across eight cities, serving around 1600 students annually. By 2022, approximately 4000 occupational therapists were practicing in diverse areas, including mental health, vocational rehabilitation, social and labor inclusion, comprehensive rehabilitation, primary care, intensive care, learning difficulties, elderly care, and support for victims of violence (Agudelo, Zúñiga, & Cristancho, 2021; Rodríguez et al., 2016).

Argentina saw the establishment of 13 occupational therapy programs, five public and eight private. A pivotal moment occurred in 1998 when the Escuela Nacional de Terapia Ocupacional (ENTO) was transferred to the National University of San Martín, resulting in the creation of five residencies and two specialties (Albino, 2022; Nabergoi, 2013; Rodríguez, 2023). By 2023, the country had approximately 12,783 occupational therapy graduates working in areas similar to those in Colombia, with an additional focus on working with incarcerated individuals and community education.

In Chile, a second program was established at the public institution Universidad de Playa Ancha in 1998. In 2002, two parallel programs were created at private universities, Universidad Mayor and Universidad Andrés Bello. By 2021, the total number of occupational therapy schools had increased to 30, offering 62 programs across 29 universities and one professional institute. About 80% of these programs are private. The degrees awarded vary by institution, including an academic degree in Bachelor of Science in Human Occupation or Bachelor of Occupational Therapy and a professional degree in occupational therapy (Avello Sáez & Fernández Orellana, 2021). In 2016, the University of Chile launched a postgraduate program, the Master in Occupation and Occupational Therapy, to address professional practice issues (Monzeli, 2019).

In Peru, two occupational therapy programs operate at the national level, and the profession is recognized in areas such as rehabilitation, assistive technology, basic education, mental health, ergonomics, and emerging fields like sports (Flores et al., 2021). Venezuela, however, faces challenges due to the lack of advanced occupational therapy training programs. Nevertheless, a sensory integration diploma program has been completed by 91 therapists from various countries, including Venezuela (Interview with Professor Virvalle Zea Segnini, 2023).

Ecuador underwent significant legislative changes that elevated its medical technology programs to the Faculty of Disability Sciences at the Central University of Ecuador, incorporating occupational therapy alongside physical and speech therapy. The University of Guayaquil established a bachelor's program, increasing the total to three public and private programs. By 2018, Ecuador had 210 occupational therapy technologists and 341 graduates. A bridging program allows previously graduated technologists to earn bachelor's degrees (CLATO, n.d.; Coello et al., 2018).

New occupational therapy programs also emerged in Panama, Uruguay, and Paraguay:

- In Panama, the Universidad de Las Américas occupational therapy program was launched in 2000. Before 2010, the field was dominated by foreign-trained professionals, but a 2010 legislative change prioritized local graduates, requiring foreign professionals to undergo a degree-leveling process. The curriculum was reformed in 2020 to include research-focused theoretical and methodological bases (Monzeli, 2021).
- Uruguay started its occupational therapy program at the Faculty of Medicine, University School of Medical Technology (EUTM), in 2001. Initially staffed by international professionals, the program evolved to meet the World Federation of Occupational Therapists (WFOT) standards. The first cohort graduated in 2009, but the bachelor's program faced setbacks, including termination of positions and a lack of program leadership (Monzeli, 2019).
- Paraguay began an occupational therapy program at Universidad Centro Médico Bautista (UCMB) in 2013, following curriculum guidelines set by the Paraguayan Association of Occupational Therapy to align with WFOT standards. Despite attempts to establish

occupational therapy programs at various universities, a lack of recognition from the Ministry of Health and limited student interest have delayed progress (Monzeli, 2019).

These developments demonstrate significant strides in occupational therapy education across Latin America, creating diverse academic and professional opportunities. However, challenges remain, including standardization of programs, access to advanced degrees, and adapting to sociopolitical contexts. The COVID-19 pandemic underscored the need for flexibility and innovation in occupational therapy education, prompting reforms and new approaches to address evolving healthcare needs (Marchant, 2021; Ortiz et al., 2023).

Influence of global and local political contexts on occupational therapy development

Political and economic shifts in the region shaped the creation and expansion of occupational therapy programs in Latin America. The neoliberal economic model, widely implemented across Latin America, promoted free market policies and reduced the state's role in regulating society and the market. This shift included the privatization of state services and increased foreign investment in sectors like banking and mining (Dávalos, 2008).

In education, these policies led to the rise of private universities and a shift in perspective from seeing citizens as "subjects of rights" to viewing them as "users" or "clients" of privately provided services. This shift often disregarded the unique needs of local communities, creating challenges for academic autonomy (Cristancho, 2021).

The 1997 WHO Conference on Health Promotion in Jakarta emphasized public policies that reorient health services toward community development, establishing "social participation" as a key principle for achieving health promotion "by and with the people" (World Health Organization, 2017). These principles transformed health systems through decentralization, promoting community involvement and citizen control. Such changes positively impacted health professions, including occupational therapy, fostering the creation of new programs and curricular revisions that integrated community-focused practices.

During this period, the profession's identity evolved from a rehabilitation and biomedical focus to a social and community-oriented approach considering each territory's social, cultural, and economic dynamics (Ramírez et al., 2022; Sotelano, 2012; Valderrama, 2019). Occupational therapists moved beyond clinical settings into community and political spaces, adapting their language and practices to include marginalized groups such as migrants, displaced people, Indigenous communities, and others. This shift reflects a move away from positivist and functionalist models toward more inclusive perspectives that aim to integrate individuals into social life (Guajardo, 2016; Valderrama, 2019).

Critical theories like "occupational therapies of the South" and decolonial and liberating theories have also emerged, advocating for models that align with the unique identity and realities of the region. Scholars like Pino Morán and Ulloa (2016) propose a critical epistemological disobedience to decolonize knowledge and incorporate Indigenous knowledge into occupational therapy education, for example the inclusion of the Guaraní language in occupational therapy training in Paraguay, enabling deeper understanding and engagement with local communities (Iaffei & Giménez, 2022).

Reflect and Discuss

- Are there emerging occupational therapy fields in your city or region beyond the health sector? What are some visible actions in these fields?
- Does the text mention specific occupational therapy actions for disease prevention?
- Are there recognizable changes in occupational therapy training programs in your country or region?
- Do you know the number and locations of universities training occupational therapists in your country or region?

The Fourth Milestone: Professional associations as a dynamic and integrative force for occupational therapy in Southern countries

Since the 1960s, pioneering countries in occupational therapy training have recognized the need to form professional associations to strengthen ties and promote development at both national and international levels. A common feature of these associations is the creation of laws to regulate professional practice. Examples include Colombia (in 1973), Argentina (in 2014), Venezuela (in 2009), and Paraguay (in 2021) (Albino, 2022; Colegio Colombiano de Terapia Ocupacional, 2020). In several Latin American countries—such as Venezuela, Peru, Paraguay, Chile, and Uruguay—professional associations have also developed documents detailing the competencies of occupational therapists, often rooted in biomedical perspectives and included in job classification manuals or health profession catalogs (Alfonso, Jaramillo, & Mora, 2023; Herrera, 2022; Trujillo, 2013; Zita, 2013).

These associations have aimed to promote the profession, highlight its value, and provide ongoing training through national and international congresses, conferences, seminars, and workshops. These events have facilitated the exchange of knowledge across Latin America, encouraging reflection, research, and the development of a more social, community-focused, and holistic approach to occupational therapy despite strong foundational paradigms (Albino, 2022; Alfonso et al., 2023; Colegio Colombiano de Terapia Ocupacional, 2020; Gómez & Imperatore, 2010; Zita, 2013).

Some countries, like Venezuela, have produced printed materials such as bulletins. In contrast, others have developed peer-reviewed journals that have enriched professional practice, such as the *Revista Argentina de Terapia Ocupacional* (Argentina), *Revista Chilena de Terapia Ocupacional* (Chile), *Revista Ocupación Humana* (Colombia), and *Cadernos Brasileiros de Terapia Ocupacional* (Brazil). These publications are well regarded in Latin America for their coverage of historical accounts, critical reflections, professional challenges, and contemporary realities (Alfonso et al., 2023).

Countries that developed the profession more recently, such as Ecuador, Paraguay, and Uruguay, are still building regulatory frameworks. Their focus has been on establishing new programs whose graduates will strengthen their profession. Nonetheless, these countries have successfully connected with regional and global occupational therapy organizations.

After establishing local associations in pioneer countries, the first international link for many was not within Latin America but through the World Federation of Occupational Therapists (WFOT). Venezuela (1968), Argentina (1970), Colombia (1976), and Chile (1980) were early members (Agudelo et al., 2021; López, 2013). By joining WFOT, these countries adopted international standards for education, occupational therapy positions, and the creation of informational bulletins, aiming to strengthen the discipline and facilitate communication among global associations. Figure 5.3 presents an overview of key milestones, affiliations, and achievements of seven occupational therapy associations in Latin America.

An early attempt to unify the region occurred in 1986 when occupational therapists from several Latin American countries attended a workshop in Lima, Peru, focused on community-based rehabilitation programs. Participants approved the creation of the Latin American Nucleus of Occupational Therapists to promote permanent communication and address shared needs. However, this initiative waned over time and did not continue beyond its initial efforts (Agudelo, 2021).

Argentinean Association of Occupational Therapists (AATO)

Founded: 1962
Key Milestones:
1963: Incorporated into health professions by the Ministry of Health
1970: Became full member of WFOT
2018: AATO branches established in 7 provinces
Affiliations: Founding member of CLATO, member of WFOT
Achievements: National Law on Professional Practice of Occupational Therapy (2006)

Venezuelan Federation of Occupational Therapists (FVTO)

Founded: 1966
Key Milestones:
1968: Full member of WFOT
1987: Established regional colleges
Affiliations: Founding member of CLATO, member of WFOT
Achievements: Approval of Occupational Therapy Practice Standards (1993)

College of Occupational Therapists of Chile (COLTOCHILE)

Founded: 1967
Key Milestones:
1980: Permanent member of WFOT
2020: Developed a national report on COVID-19 impacts
Affiliations: Founding member of CLATO, member of WFOT
Achievements: Hosted the 15th WFOT World Congress (2010)

Colombian College of Occupational Therapy (CCTO)

Founded: 1972
Key Milestones:
1988: Occupational Therapy law was established
2011: Formation of Occupational Therapy Student Network (RETO)
Affiliations: Founding member of CLATO, member of WFOT
Achievements: Bylaw reform as CCTO (2014)

Association of Occupational Therapists of Panama (ATOP)

Founded: 1985
Key Milestones:
2010: Recognized by Law 36/10
Affiliations: Member of WFOT
Achievements: Joined WFOT (2023)

Professional Association of Occupational Therapists in Peru (APTOP)

Founded: 2006
Key Milestones:
2021: Updated classification manual for Ministry of Health
Affiliations: Member of WFOT, joining CLATO in 2001
Achievements: Hosted the VIII CLATO Congress (2009)

Uruguayan Association of Occupational Therapists (AUDETO)

Founded: 2015
Key Milestones:
2017: Participated in CLATO Congress
Affiliations: In process of joining WFOT
Achievements: Documented competencies for Occupational Therapists (2017)

Figure 5.3 Key milestones and achievements of Latin American occupational therapy associations (made by Pamela Talero)

A more successful effort came a decade later when, during the III Latin American Congress of Occupational Therapy in Venezuela, representatives from Argentina, Brazil, Colombia, Chile, El Salvador, and Venezuela founded the Latin American Confederation of Occupational Therapists (CLATO). CLATO was established as a nonprofit organization to develop the profession in the region, strengthen professional identity, expand fields of action, and promote international cooperation among member associations, institutions, and professional and student organizations (Agudelo et al., 2021, p. 65).

Over time, additional countries joined CLATO, including Argentina, Bolivia, Brazil, Chile, Colombia, Costa Rica, Ecuador, Haiti, Mexico, Panama, Paraguay, Peru, Puerto Rico, the Dominican Republic, Uruguay, and Venezuela. CLATO's current mission includes promoting cohesion among member countries, disseminating achievements via social media, developing cooperation agreements to generate knowledge, and advocating for public policies to encourage the formation of new associations (Agudelo et al., 2021, p. 66).

In summary, the development of professional associations has been crucial for building a collective identity for occupational therapists in Latin America. These associations have strengthened the discipline by fostering regional and global connections and provided a platform for continuous professional growth and self-discovery (Agudelo et al., 2021).

Reflect and Discuss

- What is the relevance of being part of a local association?
- What support can the regional CLATO association provide in developing the Latin American occupational therapy profession and associations?
- Is it important to have global connections to foster regional identity?

Final reflections

The history of occupational therapy in Latin America is deeply intertwined with broader global dynamics of capitalism, colonialism, and patriarchy, where the Global South often experienced the oppressive aspirations of Global North countries. This influence extended to the intellectual development of occupational therapy, which was heavily shaped by Eurocentric and anglophone paradigms that were not always suitable for Latin American countries' cultural and social realities. The profession initially developed under a positivist framework from early 20th-century US models, emphasizing philanthropic care with female participation and mechanistic, biomedical approaches focused on neuromotor and psychiatric rehabilitation.

Over the decades, however, Latin American occupational therapy evolved in response to local needs and contexts. Shifts in political, economic, and social landscapes and international frameworks like the Alma

Ata Declaration and the Ottawa Charter spurred the development of community-based and social approaches that diverged from traditional clinical models. This led to gradually revising curricula and professional practices, integrating knowledge from various disciplines such as sociology, anthropology, and education to address complex social issues.

The expansion of occupational therapy education in Latin America from 1996 to 2022 marked a significant shift, with more private institutions entering the field, fostering competition and diversification in academic programs. The profession expanded beyond healthcare to encompass social inclusion, education, labor, and community action, driven by new concepts such as social participation, citizenship, and human rights.

Nevertheless, critical questions remain regarding the adequacy and direction of current training programs, the balance between public and private interests, and the profession's alignment with regional cultural and social identities. Additionally, the role of professional organizations like CLATO in fostering regional collaboration, advocacy, and development remains pivotal.

Conclusions

- Occupational therapy in Latin America initially developed under the hegemonic influence of Eurocentric and anglophone paradigms, which often did not align with local cultural and social contexts.
- From the 1970s onward, the profession began moving toward community-based and socially oriented models, driven by the need to address broader social determinants of health and align with WHO recommendations.
- Political instability, coups, dictatorships, and neoliberal policies affected the growth of occupational therapy programs, leading to the closure and reopening of programs and shifts in professional practice toward more community-oriented models.
- From 1996 to 2022, occupational therapy programs in Latin America grew significantly, with a notable increase in private institutions. The scope of practice also expanded beyond healthcare to include social inclusion, education, labor, and work with vulnerable populations.
- Occupational therapy organizations in Latin America, such as CLATO, have played a crucial role in advocating for professional development, promoting research, influencing public policy, and fostering regional collaboration. However, low membership and participation rates suggest a need for strategies to enhance engagement and regional identity.

Key Questions for Future Development

- Are current training programs sufficient to meet the diverse needs of each country's population?
- How should training and practice be adapted to better align with regional cultural and social identities?
- What role should private and public institutions play in shaping the profession's future?
- How can regional organizations better support professional development and advocacy in Latin America?

References

Agudelo, A., Zúñiga, S., & Cristancho, L. (2021). Perspectives and regional challenges in occupational therapy: A view from the representation of Colombia in the Latin American Confederation of Occupational Therapists – CLATO. *Revista Ocupación Humana, 21*(2), 64–71. https://doi.org/10.25214/25907816.1193

Albino, A. (2022). Formación profesional de terapistas ocupacionales de Argentina en salud mental a partir de la Ley 26.657. In A. Bottinelli, A. C. Garzón, & M. Nobergoi (Eds.), *Tramas en la Formación de Profesionales en Salud*. Editorial Teseo.

Alfonso, M. A., Jaramillo, K., & Mora, L. V. (2023). Reconstructing 50 years of the Colombian College of Occupational Therapy. *Revista Ocupación Humana, 23*(1), 41–46. https://doi.org/10.25214/25907816.1556

Araújo, M. C. (2006). *Prospectos da Democracia na América Latina em 2006*. CPDOC/FGV.

Avello Sáez, D., & Fernández Orellana, M. C. (2021). *Caracterización de la Formación de Terapeutas ocupacionales en Chile*. Comité de Calidad de Escuelas de Terapia Ocupacional de Chile.

Ayala, R. (2019). Discipline, profession and transformation. *Avances En Enfermería, 37*(3), 271–274. https://doi.org/10.15446/AV.ENFERM.V37N3.82346

Bianchi, P. C., & Malfitano, A. P. S. (2017). Formação graduada em terapia ocupacional na América Latina: Mapeando quem somos e onde estamos. *Revista de Terapia Ocupacional Da Universidade de São Paulo, 28*(2), 135. https://doi.org/10.11606/issn.2238-6149.v28i2p135-146

Biblioteca del Congreso Nacional de Chile. (2023, September 11). Chile como actor en la Guerra Fría 1973. 50 años 11 de septiembre de 1973. www.bcn.cl/conmemoracion50-septiembre-1973/guerra_fria.html

Blasier, C. (1987). *The Giant's Rival: The USSR and Latin America*. University of Pittsburgh Press.

Bottinelli, M., Nabergoi, M., Mattei, M., Díaz, F., et al. (2016). Reflections on the origins of occupational therapy training in Argentina. *Revista Ocupación Humana, 16*(2), 11–25. https://doi.org/https://doi.org/10.25214/25907816.129

CLATO. (n.d.). Historia de la terapia ocupacional en el Ecuador. Confederación Latinoamericana de Terapia Ocupacional. https://clatoterapiaocupacional.org/historia-de-la-terapia-ocupacional-en-el-ecuador

Coello, F., Chiriboga, M., & Ulloa, B. (2018). From medical technology to disability sciences. *Revista de la Facultad de Ciencias Médicas (Quito), 43*(1), 92–104. https://docs.bvsalud.org/biblioref/2019/06/1005251/9-de-la-tecnologia-medica-a-las-ciencias-de-la-discapacidad.pdf

Colegio Colombiano de Terapia Ocupacional (2020). History of the Colombian Association of Occupational Therapy. *Revista Ocupación Humana, 20*(2), 65–68. https://doi.org/10.25214/25907816.1071

Corrêa, F., & Nicacio, F. (1999). Da Institução asilar ao territorio: Caminhos para produção das intervençoes en saude. *Revista Terapia Ocupacional Universidade São Paulo, 10*(2–3), 60–68.

Cristancho, L. (2021). Characteristics of community actions of Latin American occupational therapists. *Revista Argentina de Terapia Ocupacional, 7*(1), 116–123.

Cristancho, L., & Llanos, M. (2019). Reflections on the development of occupational therapy and the professional role in three Latin American countries. *World Federation of Occupational Therapists Bulletin, 75*(2), 98–104. https://doi.org/10.1080/14473828.2019.1647988

Daneri, S. (2005). *Antecedentes de la Terapia Ocupacional en el Hospital José T. Borda: De la asunción del Dr. Domingo Cabred como director de la institución (1892) a la presencia efectiva del primer grupo de terapistas ocupacionales (1960).* Licenciatura thesis. Universidad Nacional de General San Martín.

Dávalos, P. (2008). Neoliberalismo político y estado social de derecho. *Revista Yachaikuna, 8*, 82–108.

de Oliveira, C. (2000). History of psychiatry in Venezuela: Interview with Dr. Manuel Matute. *Vitae: Academia Biomédica Digital*, no. 17, 92–96.

de Sousa Santos, B. (2018). Una nueva visión de Europa: Aprender del Sur global. In B. de Sousa Santos & José Manuel Mendes (Eds.), *Demodiversidad: Imaginar Nuevas Posibilidades Democráticas* (pp. 59–92). Ediciones Akal México.

Díaz, M. M., & Malfitano, A. P. (2021). Reflections on the idea of Latin America and its contributions to occupational therapies in the South. *Cadernos Brasileiros de Terapia Ocupacional, 29*(2568), 1–14. https://doi.org/10.1590/2526-8910.ctoen1961

Duarte, C., Fernández, A., Cruz, J., & García, S. (2016). Precursors of occupational therapy in Colombia: Subjects, institutions, occupations. *Revista Ocupación Humana, 16*(2), 93–109. https://doi.org/10.25214/25907816.140

Escobar, P., & Sepúlveda, R. (2013). *Escuela de Terapia Ocupacional Universidad de Chile: Aportes para una Historia Posible*. Universidad de Chile. https://repositorio.uchile.cl/handle/2250/151921

Flores, J., Escobar, C., Céspedes, M., Ramos, S., & García, A. (2021). Occupational therapy in Peru: A history of challenges. *Revista Herediana de Rehabilitación, 4*(1), 19–25.

García, S., Cruz, J., Duarte, C., & Fernández, A. (2022). Colombian occupational therapies: Traversing histories through a museographic exhibition. In V. Dos Santos, I. Muñoz, & M. Farias (Eds.), *Questões e Práticas Contemporâneas da Terapia Ocupacional na América do Sul* (2nd edn). Editorial CRV.

Gómez, S., & Imperatore, E. (2010). Development of occupational therapy in Latin America. *Revista de la Facultad de Medicina Universidad de Chile, 15*(12), 123–135.

Grandin, G. (2004). *The Last Colonial Massacre: Latin America in the Cold War*. University of Chicago Press.

Guajardo, A. (2016). Readings and historical accounts of occupational therapy in South America: A perspective of critical reflection. *Revista Ocupación Humana, 16*(2), 110–117. https://doi.org/10.25214/25907816.141

Herrera, J. (2022). Culture of occupational therapy in Peru: Historical and current perception. In V. Dos Santos, I. Muñoz, & M. Farias (Eds.), Questoes e praticas contemporâneas da Terapia Ocupacional na America Latina L (2nd edn., pp. 1–230). Editorial CRV.

Iaffei, F., & Giménez, L. (2022). From the Guarani land. Occupational therapy in Paraguay. In V. Dos Santos, I. Muñoz, & M. Farias (Eds.), *Questões e Práticas Contemporâneas da Terapia Ocupacional na América do Sul* (2nd edn). Editorial CRV.

Katz, C. (2015). Dualities of Latin America. *Latin American Perspectives, 42*(4), 10–42.

Laurell, A. C. (2012). Sistemas universales de salud: Retos y desafíos. Quito: Instituto Suramericano de Gobierno en Salud, Unión de Naciones Suramericanas. https://repository.unad.edu.co/bitstream/handle/10596/4830/sistemasasa.pdf

López, C. (2013). La actividad gremial nacional. In C. Forn, A. Muñoz, C. Matos, L. Castro, S. Pulido, & T. Sardi (Eds.), *Historia de la Terapia Ocupacional en Venezuela: Vol. 1* (pp. 178–191). Centro de Estudios Latinoamericanos Rómulo Gallegos.

MacDonald, A. (1972). More on the Protestant ethic. *Journal of Consulting and Clinical Psychology, 39*(1), 116.

Marchant, J. (2021). Influence of Covid-19 on the teaching role: Experience of occupational therapy teachers and students. *UCMaule, 21*(60), 76–89. https://doi.org/10.29035/ucmaule.60.76

Martínez, F. (2020). 140 years of history of Vilardebó Hospital. *Revista Uruguaya de Enfermería, 15*(2), 1–13.

Monzeli, G. (2019). *Histories of occupational therapy in Latin America: Processes of creation of the first training programs*. Doctoral thesis. Federal University of San Carlos.

Monzeli, G. A. (2021). *Histórias da Terapia Ocupacional na América Latina: A Criação dos Primeiros Programas de Formação Profissional.* João Pessoa: Editora UFPB. www.editora.ufpb.br/sistema/press5/index.php/UFPB/catalog/book/608

Monzeli, G., Morrison, R., Esquerdo, R., & Duarte, C. (2021). Histories of occupational therapy in Latin America: The first decade of the creation of professional training programs. *Revista Ocupación Humana, 21*(2), 113–136. https://doi.org/10.25214/25907816.1134

Morrison, R., Olivares, D., Graus, M., Cifuentes, D., et al. (2016). Silvia Gómez Lillo and one hundred and fifty years of occupational therapy in Chile: A biography. *Revista TOG, 13*(24), 1–27.

Mujal-León, E. (Ed.). (1989). *The USSR and Latin America: A Developing Relationship*. Taylor & Francis.

Nabergoi, M. (2013). *El proceso de transformación de la atención psiquiátrica hacia el enfoque de cuidados en salud mental en Argentina.* Doctoral thesis, National University of Lanús.

Orovitz, J. (2009). Crisis, accumulation and state form in post-neoliberal Argentina. *Memoria Académica, 5*(6), 235–253. www.memoria.fahce.unlp.edu.ar/art_revistas/pr.5115/pr.5115.pdf

Ortiz, D., Satizabal, M., Alcázar, V., Cordoba, A., & Ferrin, G. (2023). Occupational therapy in times of pandemic: Reflections from professional community practice. *Cadernos Brasileiros de Terapia Ocupacional, 31*(3419), 1–17. https://doi.org/10.1590/2526-8910.CTORE262034193

Pino Morán, J., & Ulloa, F. (2016). Perspectiva crítica desde latinoamérica: Hacia una desobediencia epistémica en terapia ocupacional contemporánea. *Cadernos de Terapia Ocupacional da UFSCar, 24*(2), 421–427.

Ramírez, D., Satizabal, M., Rojas, C., & García, S. (2022). Understandings of community in occupational therapy. *Revista Ocupación Humana, 22*(Suppl.), 102–116. https://doi.org/10.25214/25907816.1342

Ramos, F., & Castro, J. (2014). The alliance for progress in Chile and Venezuela, 1961–1963. *Tiempo y Espacio, 24*(62), 93–138. http://ve.scielo.org/scielo.php?script=sci_arttext&pid=S1315-94962014000200006&lng=es&nrm=iso&tlng=es

Rivas, A., Forn, C., Muñoz, A., Matos, C., et al. (2013). Part I History of Occupational Therapy in Venezuela. In C. Forn, A. Muñoz, C. Matos, L. Castro, S. Pulido, & T. Sardi (Eds.), *Historia de la Terapia Ocupacional en Venezuela: Vol. 1.* Centro de Estudios Latinoamericanos Rómulo Gallegos.

Rodríguez, L. (2023). The foundations and misplacements in the history of RISaM. https://risamheep.com.ar/la-residencia/historia

Rodríguez, L., Camargo, N., & Escobar, X. (2016). Occupational therapy: A historical perspective from the National University of Colombia (1966–1989). *Revista Ocupación Humana, 16*(2), 26–45. https://doi.org/10.25214/25907816.132

School of Occupational Therapy. (2023). Historia de la Escuela Terapia Ocupacional. Faculty of Medicine, University of Chile. https://medicina.uchile.cl/pregrado/resenas-escuelas/escuela-de-terapia-ocupacional

Sosa, E. (2019). Perú: La reforma educativa durante el gobierno militar de Juan Velasco Alvarado (1968–1975). *Pacarina Del Sur, 11*(42).

Sotelano, F. (2012). History of rehabilitation in Latin America. *American Journal of Physical Medicine and Rehabilitation, 91*(4), 368–373. https://doi.org/10.1097/PHM.0B013E31823CAF4A

Souza, A. D. (2012). América Latina, conceito e identidade: Algumas reflexões da história. *PRACS: Revista Eletrônica de Humanidades do Curso de Ciências Sociais da UNIFAP*, (4), 29–39.

Stucchi, S. (2015). Moral treatment and the beginnings of the madhouse in Peru. *Revista de Neuro-Psiquiatría, 78*(3), 153–153. https://doi.org/10.20453/RNP.V78I3.2573

Testa, D. (2012). Contributions to the debate on the beginnings of occupational therapy professionalization in Argentina. *Revista Chilena de Terapia Ocupacional, 12*(1), 72–87. https://doi.org/10.5354/0719-5346.2012.22054

Testa, D. (2013). Curing by doing: Poliomyelitis and the emergence of occupational therapy in Argentina, 1956–1959. *História, Ciências, Saude - Manguinhos, 20*(4), 1571–1584. https://doi.org/10.1590/S0104-59702013000500008

Trujillo, A. (1989). Perspectiva histórica sobre la disciplina de la ocupación humana. *Revista Ocupación Humana, 3*(1), 9–23.

Trujillo, A. (2002). *Terapia Ocupacional en Colombia: Vol. 1*. National University of Colombia.

Trujillo, A. (2013). Occupational therapy in Colombia continues its progress, between aspirations and achievements. *Revista Ocupación Humana, 13*(1), 5–18. https://doi.org/10.25214/25907816.19

Valderrama, C. (2019). Occupational therapies of the South: A proposal for its understanding. *Cadernos Brasileiros de Terapia Ocupacional, 27*(3), 671–680. https://doi.org/10.4322/2526-8910.ctoARF1859

World Health Organization. (2017). *Jakarta Declaration: Promoting Health*. https://apps.who.int/gb/ebwha/pdf_files/WHA51/said2.pdf

Zita, G. (2013). Part IV The International Guild Activity. In C. Forn, A. Muñoz, C. Matos, L. Castro, S. Pulido, & T. Sardi (Eds.), *Historia de la Terapia Ocupacional en Venezuela: Vol. 1* (pp. 214–250). Centro de Estudios Latinoamericanos Rómulo Gallegos.

PART 3

TERRITORIES

CHAPTER 6

Professional Training in Occupational Therapy in Latin America

TEACHING, OUTREACH, AND KNOWLEDGE PRODUCTION

Pamela Cristina Bianchi, Ricardo Lopes Correia, Carla Regina Silva, Rodolfo Morrison, Gustavo Artur Monzeli, and Beatriz Akemi Takeiti

Abstract

The first occupational therapy courses emerged in the 1950s at the technical level in Brazil, Mexico, Argentina, and Venezuela, followed by Chile and Colombia in the 1960s and Peru in the 1970s. Undergraduate training in occupational therapy is present in universities in Argentina, Bolivia, Brazil, Chile, Colombia, Costa Rica, Ecuador, El Salvador, Guatemala, Mexico, Panama, Paraguay, Peru, Puerto Rico, the Dominican Republic, Uruguay, and Venezuela, totaling more than 130 undergraduate courses in both public and private institutions. This chapter aims to present the process of training occupational therapists in Latin American countries, emphasizing teaching, outreach, and research activities at universities. Specifically, it examines how the courses are structured, their commitment to the community through university outreach, and the production of specific knowledge in and about occupational therapy in the region. This is achieved through the presentation of the group's constitution and the research developed by the Amaru Network—the Latin American Network for Knowledge Production in Occupational Therapy.

Keywords

occupational therapy; undergraduate training; knowledge production; Latin America

Learning outcomes

- Discuss the process of training occupational therapists in Latin American countries, emphasizing teaching, outreach, and research activities.
- Reflect on university outreach in the process of training in occupational therapy.
- Reflect on the production of knowledge in and about Latin American occupational therapy.
- Discuss the origins and research of the Amaru Network—the Latin American network for knowledge production in occupational therapy.

Introduction

Late industrialization and urbanization processes in Latin America in the early 1940s, the implementation of social security policies, efforts to address the effects of major epidemics, and international cooperation promoting rehabilitation programs were historical factors considered foundational for the first occupational therapy training courses in Latin American countries (Monzeli, 2021). With a technical character and assistance from foreign organizations and human resources, the profession timidly emerged in the region based on two traditional global areas: physical rehabilitation and psychiatry (Monzeli, 2021; Testa, 2012).

The first occupational therapy courses emerged in the 1950s at the technical level in Brazil, Mexico, Argentina, and Venezuela, followed by Chile and Colombia in the 1960s and Peru in the 1970s (Monzeli, 2021). The 1980s were significant for the profession, as most programs reconfigured themselves as higher education by incorporating investigative research as a requirement for course completion (Moreno, 2012).

Discussion

According to information from university websites, national associations, the Latin American Confederation of Occupational Therapists (CLATO), and field research, undergraduate training in occupational therapy is offered at universities in Argentina, Bolivia, Brazil, Chile, Colombia, Costa Rica, Ecuador, El Salvador, Guatemala, Mexico, Panama, Paraguay, Peru, Puerto Rico, the Dominican Republic, Uruguay, and Venezuela, totaling more than 130 undergraduate programs in both public and private institutions (Bianchi

& Malfitano, 2017a, 2017b). This information is presented in the Appendix to this chapter.

This chapter aims to present the process of training occupational therapists in Latin American countries, focusing on teaching, outreach, and research activities at universities.[1] Specifically, it explores how these programs are structured, their commitment to the community through university outreach, and the production of specific knowledge in and about occupational therapy in the region.

> The region had the presence of occupational therapists from the Global North, particularly British and North American professionals, who served as educators in the initial training process at various schools established in Latin American countries. Consequently, educational materials such as textbooks, lectures, and assessments were imported from different sociohistorical realities (Monzeli, 2021; Reis & Lopes, 2018). The process of incorporating and reproducing practices and theories persisted and was effective for many decades in Latin America.
>
> "...until the mid-1980s, education was based on the oral knowledge of those who invented their practice after reading one or two international manuals but learned from all kinds of demands they addressed" (Cardinalli, 2017, p. 228). After all, how could theories and practices be developed that aligned with the contexts of these countries when the profession was still adapting to the Latin American region?

Higher education in Latin America

The enslavement of Indigenous peoples, Africans, and Afro-Latinos was a tragedy of immense proportions that continues to impact deeply on culture, political systems, economies, and, hence, other sectors of society today. It is always important to emphasize that our roots are marked by domination, oppression, and unprecedented violence of one group over another, a wound that remains open (Gomes, 2019).

Besides modifying previous societies' economic, social, and cultural

1 Teaching, research, and outreach constitute the three pillars that sustain universities. Assuming that the mission of universities is to transform societies through knowledge, we can consider that the tripod of teaching, research, and outreach is the means through which this mission is accomplished. University education involves not only the transmission of knowledge in the classroom but also the development of research and the application of research findings through community outreach (Sleutjes, 1999). We will address the role of each of these activities throughout the chapter.

structures, the Spanish and Portuguese colonization also influenced the establishment of the university institution in Latin America. In Spanish-colonized countries, the university model was implemented during the colonial period, influenced by the Catholic Counter-Reformation, where the strong link between Church and State gave rise to public and Catholic institutions. These ties were later loosened during the independence processes (Cunha, 2018).

In Brazil, a country colonized by Portugal, such development did not initially exist. The absence of higher education institutions characterized the country until the 19th century (Durham, 1998). With the relocation of the monarchy's seat, the situation was reorganized, and isolated chairs were implemented to train professionals in fields such as medicine, law, and engineering (Cunha, 2018).

The public higher education model established in the 19th century has similar characteristics across Latin America that have conditioned its evolution. First, it was observed that for many years this system focused exclusively on teaching; the ideal of the university as a research center, widespread in the 19th century in economically and politically developed countries, became a late phenomenon for Latin American countries (Cunha, 2018; Durham, 1998).

According to Durham (1998), another important characteristic of the region's tradition in higher education is the belief that universities are a fundamental instrument for modernizing society, justifying state control and public funding. This conception has persisted and has been an important source of legitimacy and political projection for higher education institutions regarding resource negotiation, autonomy, and organization of academic activities.

Universities in the 20th century were organized differently in countries across the region. For example, Argentina and Mexico created large, semi-autonomous national public universities where research, when it existed, occurred in small, protected centers within schools; currently, they follow the American model with semi-autonomous research institutes and departments. In other countries like Brazil and Chile, higher education was organized among a large number of smaller institutions, both public and private, focusing on professional education with limited investments in research (Cunha, 2018).

Moving into the 21st century, the limited coverage of higher education in Latin America has become a focal point of attention in national policies across various countries, particularly regarding expanding public offerings. National projects of different formats and scopes have been designed, such as intercultural universities in the Andean region (Bolivia, Chile, Colombia,

Ecuador, Peru, and Venezuela), the expansion of federal universities in Brazil, the municipalization of higher education in Venezuela, and the establishment of national universities and regional university centers in Argentina. The expansion of university offerings has strengthened the generation of more opportunities and recognition at this level of education, directly implying the inclusion of other population groups in the academic environment (Chiroleu, 2014). Within this context, occupational therapy courses have been established and developed in the region.

Universities and the training of occupational therapists in Latin America: How are the courses organized?

Latin American students entering occupational therapy programs in the region typically take between four and ten semesters to complete their regular training. Programs lasting four to six semesters, some of which are technical in nature, are found in Puerto Rico and Venezuela. Most programs have a duration of eight to ten semesters, constituting undergraduate-level courses.

The World Federation of Occupational Therapists (WFOT), based on the Minimum Standards for the Education of Occupational Therapists, approves courses that promote the training of professionals worldwide. According to the WFOT website in Latin America, 67 courses meet these requirements and have their programs approved. These include ten courses from Argentina, 17 from Brazil, 15 from Chile, 11 from Colombia, one from Costa Rica, one from the Dominican Republic, one from Haiti, four from Mexico, one from Peru, and six from Venezuela (WFOT, 2024).

According to Bianchi and Malfitano (2017a), most courses are organized in curricular grids similar in structure, workload, and presentation of disciplines, divided into a basic cycle and a final cycle. Therefore, for example, a student entering an occupational therapy program in southern Chile will likely follow a similar educational path as a student in northeastern Brazil. Both students will study biological sciences in the early years and delve into specific occupational therapy topics in the middle to later stages of their studies.

However, it's important to note that while there are similarities in the organization of the curriculum, there are significant differences in the content covered. Studies related to the history and foundations of occupational therapy and the sociohistorical, cultural, economic, and political aspects of the countries that directly influence the profession's development are specific to each country.

Regarding the educational journey, the basic cycle encompasses the first semesters of the program. For instance, the basic cycle refers to the first two years of study in programs spanning eight to ten semesters. During this period, educational programs offer courses in biological and health sciences and social and human sciences such as psychology, exact sciences, research methods, and some specific introductory courses to occupational therapy.

Based on the analysis conducted by Bianchi and Malfitano (2017a) of the curriculum grids available on course websites, it was identified that occupational therapy programs typically include approximately 30 disciplines in their curriculum. Among these, those focused on biological sciences generally comprise biology, anatomy, physiology, neuroanatomy, neurology, pathology, immunology, psychiatry, and pharmacology. In this curriculum profile, these disciplines occupy a significant portion of the training workload compared to other areas in the basic cycle, averaging between eight and ten disciplines per course.

Courses in the humanities and social sciences are represented in smaller numbers, with approximately two disciplines per course, such as anthropology and sociology. In Brazil, many programs also include courses in the humanities that interface with the health field, such as Health and Society, and Anthropology of Health (Bianchi & Malfitano, 2017a).

The field of exact sciences also appears in small quantities, typically comprising one or two disciplines, such as applied mathematics in health and biophysics. In the Brazilian context, many programs do not include exact science disciplines, except those that propose interfaces with health, such as biostatistics. Psychology is represented by approximately two to four disciplines per course, including general psychology and developmental psychology (Bianchi & Malfitano, 2017a).

Based on Bianchi and Malfitano's analysis (2017a), disciplines related to research are relatively few, averaging about two per course, some of which are optional. Examples include research methods and scientific work methodology. On the other hand, disciplines specific to occupational therapy, which are more prevalent in the basic cycle, include fundamentals and/or history of occupational therapy, as well as therapeutic activities and resources (ART).

In the final cycle, specific occupational therapy disciplines are more numerous and are divided between theoretical and practical content. These disciplines cover various fields such as community occupational therapy, occupational therapy and primary healthcare, occupational therapy in mental health, occupational therapy in physical rehabilitation, occupational therapy in occupational health, social occupational therapy, occupational therapy and childhood, and occupational therapy and aging (Bianchi & Malfitano, 2017a).

It is important to note that some courses have unique curriculum structures due to methodological choices and/or institutional pedagogical projects. For instance, the occupational therapy program at the Federal University of Sergipe in Brazil adopts active learning methodologies in annual cycles divided by competencies, aiming for the generalist training of occupational therapists (Hiratuka et al., 2014).

Similarly, the Federal University of São Paulo in Brazil organizes its curriculum into four training axes (Human Being in its Biological Dimension, Human Being and its Social Insertion, Work in Health, and Approach to Specific Practice), emphasizing interdisciplinary and integrated education across six courses: occupational therapy, psychology, nutrition, physiotherapy, physical education, and social work (Jurdi et al., 2018).

Based on analysis by Bianchi and Malfitano (2017b), it's evident that occupational therapy courses in Latin American universities have similar structures and areas of focus, with a strong emphasis on the biological and health fields, indicating a significant biomedical influence in their education and noticeable gaps in the teaching of social and human sciences.

These findings align with the results of research conducted by Pan and Lopes (2019) on Brazilian federal universities. Their investigation revealed a high percentage of content oriented toward biological and health sciences, with a disproportionate representation compared to social and human sciences. Pan and Lopes attribute this to the profession's historical roots, which in the 1960s underwent a movement toward aligning with the assumptions of the biomedical model to achieve technical and scientific validation. The implications of this process are still visible today in the quest for professional legitimacy and identity construction.

It is crucial to understand that this period was marked by the implementation of a privatization policy, with incentives for hospital-centric institutions in psychiatric care, for example, amidst the period of military dictatorship (1964–1985) characterized by censorship and violence of a totalitarian state. During this time, occupational therapy was heavily subjected to medical knowledge and power (Cardinalli, 2022).

The discussion about the adoption of the biomedical model in education and, subsequently, in professional practice extends beyond the offering of biological science disciplines. It encompasses its impact on the adopted professional conduct. Nonetheless, it serves as objective data to support discussions about predominant education and orientations in the field.

It is evident from the information on the educational journey in the region that the field of health, from a biomedical perspective, remains a priority theme in graduate education in occupational therapy in Latin America. However, there is a need to question the historical characteristics and the emergence of new social issues in the region and the actual preparedness of professionals to deal with interventions tailored to the Latin American context, which demands professionals engaged with their social reality (Bianchi & Malfitano, 2017b).

According to Galheigo et al. (2018), "[t]he emergence of critical thinking in Brazilian occupational therapy stands out in the late 1970s, initially through criticism of hegemonic practices, and subsequently through propositions of emancipatory practices" (p. 734). The authors acknowledge that the period from the late 1970s to 1996 was marked by the problematization of knowledge and practices in occupational therapy, drawing from collective health and human and social sciences. The period between 1997 and 2005 was related to the expansion and differentiation of fields of investigation, knowledge, and practices in occupational therapy, with sociopolitical contextualization, theoretical-conceptual problematization, and propositions of emancipatory practices from/for/with singular and collective experiences involving human activity and daily life (Galheigo et al., 2018).

This brief contextualization reinforces the debate on the importance of conceptual foundations related to human and social sciences and the arts and how they imply the theoretical-methodological production of occupational therapeutic knowledge and practices. It represents a critical and responsible dimension, engaging in ethical-political commitment in occupational therapy practice. This theoretical contribution fosters contextualized reflections on the real demands and needs of individuals and collectives in their daily lives, perpetuated by explorations, violations, and inequalities of hegemonic processes. As Silvestrini, Silva, and Almeida Prado (2019) describe,

> occupational therapists can contribute to the production of strategies, reflections, and practices that are anti-hegemonic, anti-colonial, anti-heterocispatriarchal, and anti-racist in the pursuit of disrupting and overcoming the impacts generated by hegemonic and violent practices in ways of life and human relationships. (p. 934)

University outreach, commitment to the community, and occupational therapy

According to Paulo Freire (1988), university outreach means to educate oneself in the practice of freedom; in other words, it is a dialogical educational practice that

> is the task of those who know that they know little—hence they know that they know something and can thus come to know more—in dialogue with those who almost always think they know nothing, so that these individuals,

> by transforming their thinking that they know nothing into knowing that they know little, can equally come to know more. (Freire, 1988, p. 15)

In other words, university outreach consists of activities that, coupled with teaching and research, disseminate the knowledge generated by the university, bringing it closer to society (Sleutjes, 1999) and often revisiting and transforming that knowledge alongside it. In this way, it promotes the interrelation between university and society, serving as a tool for reflection and democratization of academic knowledge through exchanging knowledge and dialogues with communities (Figueiredo et al., 2022).

Although widely used in Latin American countries, university outreach originated in England in the second half of the 19th century. In the form of courses for adults, akin to continuing education, English professors would leave their universities to teach subjects such as literature, history, physical sciences, and political sciences to a public seeking information and knowledge for practical application and/or reflection on themes relevant to their everyday lives (Paula, 2013).

According to Paula (2013), university outreach is a product of a specific moment in history when the effective imposition of capitalist production exacerbated contradictions experienced by the working class, who, subjected to capital, sought to understand, denounce the capitalist social order, and seek alternatives to their ways of life, such as socialism.

An important historical milestone for university outreach in Latin America was the Reform of Córdoba (1918), considered a process of university restructuring that emerged from a university student manifestation recognizing the university regime as "anachronistic," outdated for its time, and unsuitable as monastic and monarchical structures were surpassed, advocating for a more democratic university (Azevedo, Braggio, & Catani, 2018). This movement sparked numerous debates and events that continue to influence the meanings and significance of outreach in the region, including current debates on implementing outreach as a mandatory part of the curricula of all higher-education courses.

It was through the work of Paulo Freire at the University of Recife in Brazil that the effective integration between the university and the community was concretized. It was through the pedagogue's questioning and practices that the university discovered and developed "instruments that bring it closer to the popular sectors, both through concrete literacy actions and through the development of methodologies for interaction between technical-scientific knowledge and popular cultures" (Paula, 2013, p. 17).

In practical terms, nowadays, outreach activities have enabled a closer integration of theory and practice within real contexts and have facilitated the training of professionals sensitive to the plurality of individuals and population groups and to social and cultural diversity through critical and active reflection in the onsite teaching-learning process (Figueiredo & Paterra, 2019).

Furthermore, university outreach can contribute to the formulation and development of various policies, either through its practical actions or through its integration with teaching and research, strengthening spaces for dialogue among different sectors of society and fulfilling the social commitment of the university (Forproex, 2012).

Reflect and Discuss

Did you know that, in Brazil, outreach activities are part of the workload for students to complete?

According to current Brazilian guidelines for outreach in higher education, interventions directly involving communities outside higher education institutions and linked to student training are considered outreach activities. These activities, categorized as programs, projects, courses and workshops, events, and service provision, must be included in the curriculum of undergraduate courses and comprise at least 10% of the total student curriculum workload, in a process referred to as the curricularization of outreach (Brasil, 2018).

Due to the theoretical and practical nature of the disciplines and knowledge offered in the field of occupational therapy in Brazil, there have been numerous outreach activities. Typically, outreach is coordinated by university faculty and conducted by a team comprising faculty members, students, and members of the participating communities.

According to Figueiredo et al. (2022), 43 publications have characterized research data and experience reports on outreach projects in the country's universities through a scoping review of university outreach in Brazilian occupational therapy. These projects span various fields of action, target different age groups and locations, and employ diverse working methodologies, such as workshops and/or individual follow-ups.

For example, Joaquim et al. (2014) documented the experiences of a group of mothers of hospitalized infants aimed at providing support, guidance, and information on infant care during and after hospitalization, reorganizing daily life, and addressing anxieties and fears during the hospitalization period. On the other hand, Correia and Akerman (2015) described an interdisciplinary experience in participatory local development; the group conducted social assistance, health, and environmental education activities within a riverside community in Brazil, aiming to strengthen their community relations.

It is worth noting that outreach projects also significantly contribute to research development in occupational therapy. Through outreach, it becomes possible to establish study fields to advance theoretical-practical discussions, systematize experiences, and build methodological frameworks to support the development of research that enhances occupational therapy.

Knowledge production and research in Latin American occupational therapy

In the last axis of the teaching-outreach-research tripod, universities have another important role: the commitment to producing knowledge that contributes to and addresses the demands of everyday life. In occupational therapy courses in Latin American countries, it is common to develop research as part of the educational process, often referred to as final undergraduate projects. Additionally, there are postgraduate programs, including master's and doctoral courses, focused on specific knowledge production in occupational therapy in Brazil, Chile, Colombia, and Mexico (Bianchi & Malfitano, 2017a, 2017b).

We recognize that there are many ways and different places to produce knowledge; the university is just one of them. It is important to highlight that knowledge is being produced in communities and territories by social movements, identity collectives, traditional peoples, and many others. Thus, we understand that all knowledge production is governed by a series of dimensions that interfere with and determine the studies, themes, conditions, and relationships for research development. These include geographical location, social, political, and economic context, hegemonies present in modern science, disputes over knowledge and areas of expertise, and political positioning, among many others.

In this context, the Amaru Network[2] constitutes a collaborative network for producing and disseminating knowledge in occupational therapy, whether produced within universities by faculty and students or in practice settings by occupational therapists and their partner groups and communities.

2 Amaru, a majestic serpent revered by the ancient Inca culture, embodies profound wisdom and boundless learning. It symbolizes not just the principle of organization and regeneration of life, but also represents the exquisite process of birth, the incredibly potent force that ignites creation in all its forms. Above all, it stands as a poignant symbol and metaphor of relentless self-renewal of knowledge, continuously reshaping and revitalizing the landscapes of understanding and wisdom.

Amaru Network—the Latin American network for knowledge production in occupational therapy

In 2017, during the I Mexican Congress of Occupational Therapy and XII Latin American Congress of Occupational Therapy "History, Present, and Vision of Occupational Therapy in Latin America," held in Mexico City, a group of occupational therapists from Brazil, Chile, and Argentina, sensitive to the debate on knowledge production in occupational therapy, gathered to foster a network to produce and disseminate knowledge specific to the Latin American region in occupational therapy.

This group of professionals and friends remained organized to structure the Amaru Network. In 2018, its creation was officially announced during the 1st International Encounter of Occupational Therapies from the South in Santiago, Chile. The following year, its launch occurred during the X Argentine Congress and XIII Latin American Congress of Occupational Therapy in Tucumán, Argentina. During these events, aspirations, ethical considerations, and methods for producing and disseminating occupational therapy knowledge specific to the region were shared, as well as their place within the global and international landscape of the field.

Since then, the Amaru Network has been actively developing collective strategies to:

- map occupational therapists across the region
- identify the types of knowledge being produced
- develop methods for collective production and dissemination of knowledge
- engage in dialogue within the global and international arena of the field, (re)shaping linguistic structures
- enhance communication with society about occupational therapy as a social right to effectively address the complex demands of social reality.

As described by Lopes et al. (2023),

> we see this collective and movement as a political-epistemic category that can serve to designate and guide counter-hegemonic processes of production and dissemination of knowledge in occupational therapy, and to establish other truths situated in the scientific and cosmological reality of the Latin American region. (p. 134)

We understand the importance of this position based on three proposition axes: (a) to identify, map, share, produce, and disseminate specific knowledge in occupational therapy from Latin America, which allows for the institutionalization of a strong and reliable scientific discipline of knowledge; (b) to transfer knowledge produced in occupational therapy to other disciplines; and (c) to promote the political-epistemic defense and discourse of occupational therapy as a social right for diverse individuals, groups, and populations that call for the area to position itself politically and ethically and to make sociotechnical decisions for increasingly complex societal demands (Lopes Correia et al., 2022).

As the first initiative of this network, the group conducted a comprehensive mapping, via online form, of research and researchers in occupational therapy across Latin America. The study aimed to map and analyze the profiles of researchers, study topics, research groups, types of studies, dissemination of produced knowledge, and collaboration networks in occupational therapy in Latin America. The mapping sought to highlight researchers who are building knowledge in/for occupational therapy, aiming to contribute to strengthening the professional ties between countries and the scientific production of the profession in the region. We will now present some of the information found.

Amaru mapping: Research and researchers in occupational therapy in Latin America

The mapping obtained 108 responses from occupational therapists across nine different countries. The highest concentration of responses came from Brazil (n = 54), followed by Chile (n = 21), Colombia (n = 19), Argentina (n = 9), Costa Rica (n = 1), Ecuador (n = 1), Guatemala (n = 1), Panama (n = 1), and Uruguay (n = 1).

Regarding the professions of the collaborators, 73 are educators, 58 work as occupational therapists, 52 are researchers, six are occupational therapy students, four are *stricto sensu* postgraduate students, three responded "other," and one responded with a *lato sensu* postgraduate degree. Concerning postgraduate education, 33 collaborators completed an academic master's degree, 55 completed a professional master's degree, and 58 pursued doctoral research.

The mapping questioned its participants: What do you understand as knowledge in occupational therapy? The responses were open-ended and showed us that most participants (n = 101) consider the object of occupational therapy (occupation, activity, daily life) as knowledge. This was followed by 97 participants who believe that knowledge arises from practice in occupational therapy; 41 people consider it as academic study in occupational therapy; 23 mention academic research; 19 discuss production articulated with the populations, collectives, and social movements; eight mention the political dimension of occupational therapy; and finally, two consider it as undergraduate and postgraduate professional training. Six people did not respond.

Regarding the type of knowledge that participants produce in and for occupational therapy, 92 consider scientific research, 48 consider political knowledge as a juridical-institutional instrument, 33 consider political knowledge as a social movement, 14 consider aesthetic-artistic-cultural knowledge, 16 mention other types of knowledge not present in the form options, and only two do not consider that they produce knowledge in and for occupational therapy. Five people did not respond.

A significant number of occupational therapists state that they conduct research in groups (such as professional associations, study groups, and social movements, among others), either institutional or specific to occupational therapy (n = 36) or composed of professionals from different areas (n = 53). Another group states that they develop knowledge within communities of practice (n = 11), while others work with non-institutional occupational therapy groups (n = 16), or with professionals from other areas (n = 11). Some colleagues (n = 17) indicated that they build knowledge alongside social movements outside academic institutions.

The mapping also sought to understand the main topics studied by Latin American occupational therapists. Regarding major knowledge areas, we found that 39% of the collaborators research occupational therapy; another 36% study health topics; and 20% focus their research on humanities and social sciences as well as arts; 5% did not respond.

Regarding the main themes studied, the following were indicated: occupational therapy fundamentals (n = 44), education (n = 30), public health (n = 25), art and culture (n = 23), rights and public policies (n = 22), mental health (n = 22), disabilities (n = 21), childhood (n = 20), rehabilitation (n = 16), community area (n = 12), social area (n = 11), elderly (n = 11), work (n = 10), gender and sexuality (n = 9), alcohol and other drugs (n = 5), along with many other freely mentioned topics. Table 6.1 provides examples of the topics studied by occupational therapists within these themes.

Table 6.1 Themes investigated by Latin American occupational therapists

Themes	Examples of topics studied
Fundamentals of occupational therapy	Histories of occupational therapy; occupational therapy education; occupational therapy knowledge and skills
Education	Inclusive education; public school; higher education
Public health	Primary healthcare; epidemiology; health promotion
Art and culture	Artistic and bodily practices; popular cultures; cultural accessibility; interculturality

Rights and public policies	Human rights; public policy analysis
Mental health	Mental health care processes; psychosocial care and mental health
Disabilities	Inclusion of people with disabilities; rights of people with disabilities; accessibility
Childhood	Child development; play
Rehabilitation	Physical rehabilitation; hand rehabilitation
Community area	Community occupational therapy; community intervention
Social area	Social occupational therapy; social field
Elderly	Gerontology; aging; elderly health
Work	Work inclusion; ergonomics; solidarity economy
Gender and sexuality	LGBTQI+ population, gender, and family; dissident sexualities
Alcohol and other drugs	Harm reduction; chemical dependency
Other topics	Sensory integration; validation of assessment tools; assistive technology; territory; Black population; urban planning; sports; hospital setting; alternative communication

It is interesting to note that the majority of collaborators dedicate themselves to producing knowledge within the field of occupational therapy, conducting studies on the histories and identities in their countries, reflecting on undergraduate education and what is specific to occupational therapy knowledge and skills, such as their objects of study: occupation, daily life, and activity.

While what has been produced by occupational therapists is highly relevant to the field, the mapping showed us that the circulation of their work happens more within their own countries, nationally (n = 46), or within their states and cities (n = 24). Twenty-three colleagues indicated that their studies circulate in journals from other countries. At the same time, nine reported maintaining their productions only at an individual level, and six were unsure about this.

We acknowledge that this is not a comprehensive overview of occupational therapists producing knowledge in the Latin American region; it merely provides some insights into the paths guiding the interests and investments of our colleagues. A documentary investigation would be necessary to obtain a general overview of formal research groups in the sample countries. However, it is known that each country has a specific way of organizing its research groups; for example, in Brazil, there is the Directory of Research Groups of the National Council for Scientific and Technological

Development, which gathers information about research groups at Brazilian universities. The dissemination of this information poses a challenge for this discussion and points to the need to concentrate this information to encourage and facilitate communication among groups/researchers.

Conclusions

- Undergraduate programs in occupational therapy in Latin America have focused on constructing a formative path based on the tripod of teaching, research, and outreach. In addition to classroom activities and within university walls, graduates in occupational therapy in the region also gain formative experiences with the external community through university outreach activities and research development.
- Expanding community-based, engaged, and critical education is directly linked to integrated education, research, and outreach, which depend on institutions with greater structure, autonomy, incentives, and commitment to educational, cultural, and social transformation.
- Although discussions on social, cultural, and community fields are prominent in the Latin American region, there is still an absence or insufficiency of content from social sciences, humanities, and arts that could promote greater problem-solving capacity, critical awareness, and expansion of fields of action.
- The mapped information on the knowledge production of Latin American occupational therapists has indicated greater investment in reflections on local and contextual characteristics of the field in the region, demonstrating progress toward recognition of one or several occupational therapies.
- The number of occupational therapy training programs has grown in the last two decades. However, the number of professional occupational therapists is still insufficient to meet population demands, especially regarding public policies. Some countries lack undergraduate occupational therapy programs, and some have only one.
- Training in research at the master's and doctoral levels in occupational therapy remains challenging. Nevertheless, significant experiences are observed, such as in Brazil, which has had a master's program since 2010 and the only doctoral program in occupational therapy since 2014 at the Federal University of São Carlos.
- Although hegemonic discourses, practices, and frameworks are also reinforced in the region, there is an ongoing process of significant rupture with processes of reproduction, which has a unique capacity

to autonomously promote new debates, practices, experiences, perspectives, and modes of knowledge in occupational therapy, associated with the Latin American dimension and the diverse realities and contexts specific to each place.

References

Azevedo, M. L. N., Braggio, A. K., & Catani, A. M. (2018). A Reforma Universitária de Córdoba de 1918 e sua influência no Brasil: Um foco no movimento estudantil antes do golpe de 1964. [The Córdoba University Reform of 1918 and its influence in Brazil: A focus on the student movement before the 1964 coup.] *Revista Latinoamericana de Educación Comparada, 13*(9), 37–51.

Bianchi, P. C., & Malfitano, A. P. S. (2017a). Formação graduada em terapia ocupacional na América Latina: Mapeando quem somos e onde estamos [Graduate training in occupational therapy in Latin America: Mapping who we are and where we are]. *Revista de Terapia Ocupacional da Universidade de São Paulo, 28*(2), 135–146.

Bianchi, P. C., & Malfitano, A. P. S. (2017b). Formación en terapia ocupacional en América Latina: ¿Avanzamos hacia la cuestión social? [Occupational therapy education in Latin America: Are we moving to the social issue?] *World Federation of Occupational Therapists Bulletin, 73*(1), 15–23.

Brasil. (2018). *Resolução nº 7, de 18 de dezembro de 2018. Diretrizes para a Extensão na Educação Superior Brasileira* [Guidelines for Outreach in Brazilian Higher Education]. Diário Oficial [da] República Federativa do Brasil, Brasília, seção 1, 49.

Cardinalli, I. (2022). *Ninho de nós: Sentidos da atividade humana em terapia ocupacional.* Doctoral thesis, Federal University of São Carlos. https://repositorio.ufscar.br/handle/ufscar/15866

Chiroleu, A. (2014). Democratización universitaria y desigualdad social en América Latina [University democratization and social inequality in Latin America]. *Política Universitária (Buenos Aires, Argentina), 1*(1), 26–31.

Correia, R., & Akerman, M. (2015). Desenvolvimento local participativo, rede social de suporte e ocupação humana: Relato de experiência em projeto de extensão [Participatory local development, social network support, and human occupation: Experience report in an outreach project]. *Revista de Terapia Ocupacional da Universidade de São Paulo, 26*(1), 159–165.

Cunha, C. (2018). Educação na América Latina: Pressupostos e alcance de estudos comparativos [Education in Latin America: Assumptions and scope of comparative studies]. *Revista Lusófona de Educação, 41*, 153–174. https://doi.org/10.24140/issn.1645-7250.rle41.10

Durham, E. R. (1998). O ensino superior na América latina: Tradições e tendências [Higher education in Latin America: Traditions and trends]. *Novos Estudos CEBRAP, 51*, 91–105.

Figueiredo, M. O., Batistão, R., Silva, C. R., Martinez, C. M. S., & Roiz, R. G. (2022). A atividade de extensão na terapia ocupacional: Revisão de escopo na literatura nacional [University outreach in occupational therapy: Scoping review in Brazilian literature]. *Cadernos Brasileiros de Terapia Ocupacional, 30*, e2908. https://cadernosdeto.ufscar.br/index.php/cadernos/article/view/2908

Figueiredo, M. O., & Paterra, I. P. (2019). As atividades de extensão e a formação em terapia ocupacional: Percepção docente [Extension activities and training in occupational therapy: Teacher perception]. In C. R. Silva (Ed.), *Atividades Humanas e Terapia Ocupacional: Saber-Fazer, Cultura, Política e Outras Resistências* [Human activities and occupational therapy: Know-how, culture, politics and other resistances] (pp. 314–340). São Paulo: Hucitec Editora.

Forproex (Fórum de Pró-Reitores de Extensão das Universidades Públicas Brasileiras). (2012). *Política Nacional de Extensão Universitária* [National University Outreach Policy]. MEC/SeSU.

Freire, P. (1988). *Extensão ou Comunicação?* [Outreach or Communication?] (10th edn.). São Paulo: Paz e Terra.

Galheigo, S. M., Braga, C. P., Arthur, M. A., & Matsuo, C. M. (2018). Produção de conhecimento, perspectivas e referências teórico-práticas na terapia ocupacional brasileira: Marcos e tendências em uma linha do tempo [Knowledge production, perspectives, and theoretical-practical references in Brazilian occupational therapy: Milestones and tendencies in a timeline]. *Cadernos Brasileiros De Terapia Ocupacional, 26*(4), 723–738. https://doi.org/10.4322/2526-8910.ctoAO1773

Gomes, L. (2019). Escravidão: do primeiro leilão de cativos em Portugal à morte de Zumbi dos Palmares [Slavery: from the first auction of captives in Portugal to the death of Zumbi dos Palmares]. Globo Livros: Rio de Janeiro, Brasil.

Hiratuka, E., Duque, A. M., Andrade, F. L., Silva, M. N. S., Menta, A. S., & Soares, T. B. A. (2014). Metodologias ativas como estratégias de ensino: Experiência da terapia ocupacional na UFS [Active methodologies as teaching strategies: Experience of occupational therapy at UFS]. *Cadernos de Terapia Ocupacional da UFSCar, 22*(Suppl.), 487–492.

Joaquim, R. H. V. T., Silvestrini, M. S., & Marini, B. P. R. (2014). Grupo de mães de bebês prematuros hospitalizados: Experiência de intervenção de terapia ocupacional no contexto hospitalar [Group of mothers of hospitalized premature newborns: Experience of occupational therapy intervention in hospital context]. *Cadernos de Terapia Ocupacional da UFSCar, 22*(1), 145–150.

Jurdi, A, P. S., Nicolau, S. M., Figueiredo, L. R. U., Rossit, R. A. S., Maximino, V. S., & Borba, P. L. O. (2018). Revisitar processos: Revisão da matriz curricular do curso de terapia ocupacional da Universidade Federal de São Paulo [Revisit processes: Review of the curricular matrix of the occupational therapy course at the Federal University of São Paulo]. *Interface (Botucatu), 22*(65), 527–538.

Lopes Correia, R., Silva, C. R., Bianchi, P. C., Monzeli, G. A., et al. (2023). Amaru: Rede de conhecimento em terapia ocupacional da América Latina [Amaru: Knowledge network in occupational therapy in Latin America]. *Groupwork, 31*(1–2), 130–160. https://doi.org/10.1921/gpwk.v30i3.1709

Monzeli, G. A. (2021). *Histórias da Terapia Ocupacional na América Latina: A Criação dos Primeiros Programas de Formação Profissional* [Histories of Occupational Therapy in Latin America: The Creation of the First Professional Training Programs]. João Pessoa, Brazil Editora UFPB.

Moreno, A. F. (2012). Publicaciones seriadas de la terapia ocupacional en Latinoamerica [Serial publications on occupational therapy in Latin America]. *Cadernos de Terapia Ocupacional da UFSCar, 20*(2), 287–292.

Pan, L. C., & Lopes, R. E. (2019). La enseñanza de la terapia ocupacional social en las instituciones federales de educación superior en Brasil [The teaching of social occupational therapy in federal institutions of higher education in Brazil]. *Revista Chilena de Terapia Ocupacional, 19*(1), 23–34.

Paula, J. A. (2013). A extensão universitária: História, conceito e propostas [University outreach: History, concept, and proposals]. *Interfaces – Revista de Extensão da UFMG, 1*(1), 5–23.

Reis, S. C. C. A. G., & Lopes, R. E. (2018). O início da trajetória de institucionalização acadêmica da terapia ocupacional no Brasil: O que contam os(as) docentes pioneiros(as) sobre a criação dos primeiros cursos [The beginning of the trajectory of occupational therapy academic institutionalization in Brazil: What pioneer professors tell about the creation of the first courses]. *Cadernos Brasileiros De Terapia Ocupacional, 26*(2), 255–270.

Silvestrini, M. S., Silva, C. R., & Almeida Prado, A. C. S. (2019). Terapia ocupacional e cultura: Dimensões ético-políticas e resistências [Occupational therapy and culture: Ethical-political dimensions and resistances]. *Cadernos Brasileiros De Terapia Ocupacional, 27*(4), 929–940. https://doi.org/10.4322/2526-8910.ctoARF1727

Sleutjes, M. H. S. C. (1999). Refletindo sobre os três pilares de sustentação das universidades: Ensino-pesquisa-extensão [Reflecting on the three support pillars of universities: Teaching-research-outreach]. *Revista De Administração Pública, 33*(3), 99–101.

Testa, D. (2012). Aportes para el debate sobre los inicios de la profesionalización de la terapia ocupacional en Argentina [Contributions to the debate on the beginnings of the professionalization of occupational therapy in Argentina]. *Revista Chilena de Terapia Ocupacional, 12*(1), 72–87. https://doi.org/10.5354/0719-5346.2012.22054

WFOT (World Federation of Occupational Therapy). (2024). WFOT Approved Education Programmes. https://wfot.org/programmes/education/wfot-approved-education-programmes

Appendix

Undergraduate programs in occupational therapy at Latin American higher education institutions[1]

Country	Higher Education Institution
Argentina	Universidad de Buenos Aires (UBA)
	Universidad Nacional de San Martín (UNSAM)
	Universidad Nacional de Villa María (UNVM)
	Universidad Nacional de La Rioja (UNLaR)
	Universidad Nacional de Mar del Plata (UNMdP)
	Universidad Nacional de Quilmes (UNQ)
	Universidad Nacional del Litoral (UNL)
	Universidad de Chubut (UDC)
	Universidad del Salvador (USal)
	Universidad Abierta Americana (UAI) – Rosario
	Universidad Abierta Americana (UAI) – Buenos Aires
	Universidad Católica de La Plata (UCALP)
	Pontificia Universidad Católica Argentina
	Universidad del Norte Santo Tomás de Aquino (UNSTA)
	Universidad Nacional Juan Agustín Maza (UMaza)
	Universidad Católica de Córdoba
	Universidad Católica de Salta
	Universidad Católica de Cuyo
	Universidad Católica de Santa Fé
	ISalud
	Universidad Gastón Dachary

cont.

1 The information presented in the table is for the year 2024. It is important to note that, in the region, courses often open and/or close. Therefore, the data provided are subject to variations depending on the temporal context in which they are consulted.

Country	Higher Education Institution
Brazil	Escola Superior da Amazônia (ESAMAZ)
	Universidade da Amazônia (UNAMA)
	Universidade do Estado do Pará (UEPA)
	Universidade Federal do Pará (UFPA)
	Centro Universitário Aparício Carvalho (FIMCA)
	Faculdade Martha Falcão (FMF Wyden)
	Universidade de Brasília
	Faculdade União de Goyazes (FUG)
	Universidade Federal do Paraná (UFPR)
	Faculdade de Ensino Superior de São Miguel do Iguaçu (FAESI)
	Associação Catarinense de Ensino Guilherme Guimbala (FGG)
	Universidade Federal de Santa Maria - UFSM
	Universidade Federal de Pelotas - UFPel
	Centro Universitário da Serra Gaúcha - FSG
	Universidade Estadual de Ciências da Saúde de Alagoas - UNCISAL
	Universidade Federal da Paraíba (UFPB)
	Centro Universitário UniFACID Wyden
	Universidade Federal de Pernambuco (UFPE)
	Universidade Federal de Sergipe (UFS)
	Universidade Estadual do Ceará (UECE)
	Universidade Federal de Minas Gerais (UFMG)
	Universidade Federal do Triângulo Mineiro (UFTM)
	Universidade Federal do Espírito Santo (UFES)
	Instituto Federal de Educação, Ciência e Tecnologia do Rio de Janeiro (IFRJ)
	Universidade Federal do Rio de Janeiro (UFRJ)
	Centro Universitário Saúde ABC (FMABC)
	Pontifícia Universidade Católica de Campinas (PUC-CAMP)
	Universidade de São Paulo (USP) - São Paulo
	Universidade de São Paulo (USP) - Ribeirão Preto
	Universidade de Sorocaba (UNISO)
	Universidade Estadual Paulista Júlio de Mesquita Filho (UNESP)
	Universidade Federal de São Carlos (UFSCar)
	Universidade Federal de São Paulo (UNIFESP)
	Centro Universitário Claretiano (CEUCLAR)
	Universidade Paranaense
	Centro Universitário de Barra Mansa (UBM)

	Universidade Federal da Bahia (UFBA)
	Universidade de Pernambuco (UPE)
	Faculdades Integradas de Três Lagoas (AEMS)
	Centro Universitário Ingá (UNINGÁ)
	Faculdade Uniguaçu (UNIGUAÇU)
	Centro Universitário Fatecie (UNIFATECIE)
Bolivia	Universidad Mayor de San Andrés
Chile	Universidad de Chile
	Universidad de los Andes
	Universidad de Playa Ancha
	Universidad de Antofagasta
	Universidad de las Américas
	Universidad de La Frontera
	Universidad de Magallanes
	Universidad SEK
	Universidad del Desarrollo
	Universidad Austral de Chile (Isla Teja)
	Universidad de Santiago de Chile
	Universidad Santo Tomás
	Universidad de Talca
	Universidad Andrés Bello
	Universidad San Sebastián
	Universidad Mayor
	Universidad Autónoma de Chile
	Universidad Autónoma de Chile – Santiago
	Universidad Central de Chile
	Universidad Católica de Temuco
	Universidad Bernardo O'Higgins – Santiago
	Universidad Viña del Mar
	Universidad Católica del Maule (UCM)
	Universidad de O'Higgins – Rancagua
	Universidad Academia de Humanismo Cristiano
	Universidad de los Lagos – Puerto Montt
	Universidad de los Lagos – Chiloé
	Universidad Católica
	Universidad Central Región de Coquimbo
	Universidad Católica del Maule

cont.

Country	Higher Education Institution
Colombia	Escuela Colombiana de Rehabilitación
	Universidad de Santander
	Universidad Manuela Beltrán – Bucaramanga
	Universidad Manuela Beltrán – Bogotá
	Universidad Nacional de Colombia
	Universidad de Pamplona
	Universidad Colegio Mayor de Nuestra Señora del Rosário
	Universidad del Valle
	Universidad Mariana de Pasto
	Universidad Metropolitana
Costa Rica	Universidad Santa Paula
Equador	Universidad Central del Ecuador
	Universidad LAICA Eloy Alfaro de Manabí
Guatemala	Universidad de San Carlos de Guatemala
Haiti	Université Episcopale d'Haïti
Mexico	Centro de Rehabilitacion "Gaby Brimer"
	Centro Mexicano Universitario de Ciencias y Humanidades
	Centro de Rehabilitación y Educación Especial Puebla
	Instituto Científico de Educación Superior
	Instituto Mexicano del Seguro Social
	Instituto Nacional de Rehabilitación
	Instituto Teleton de Estudios Superiores en Rehabilitacion
	Instituto de Terapia Ocupacional
	Universidad Autónoma del Estado de México
Panama	Universidad Especializada de las Américas
Paraguay	Universidad Centro Médico Bautista
Peru	Universidad Nacional Mayor de San Marcos
Puerto Rico	Universidad de Puerto Rico – Humacao
	Universidad de Puerto Rico – Recinto de Ciencias Médicas
	Universidad Interamericana
	Huertas College – Caguas
Dominican Republic	Universidad Catolica Santo Domingo (UCSD)
Uruguay	Universidad de la Republica Uruguay

Venezuela	Colegio Universitário de los Teques Cecílio Acosta
	Colegio Universitário de Rehabilitación May Hamilton
	Universidad Central de Venezuela
	Universidad Politécnica Territorial de los Altos Mirandinos "Cecilio Acosta"
	Universidad Politécnica Territorial del Norte de Monagas "Ludovico Silva"
	Universidad Territorial Deltana "Francisco Tamayo"
	Universidad Nacional Experimental "Rómulo Gallegos"
	Universidad de las Ciencias de la Salud "Hugo Rafael Chávez Frías" núcleo Bolívar
	Universidad de las Ciencias de la Salud "Hugo Rafael Chávez Frías" núcleo Anzoategui
	Universidad de las Ciencias de la Salud "Hugo Rafael Chávez Frías" núcleo La Guaira
	Universidad Nacional Experimental "Francisco de Miranda"

CHAPTER 7

Human Movements in Latin America and the Caribbean

APPROACHES FOR OCCUPATION-BASED INTERVENTIONS

Julián Samacá Pulido and Pamela Talero Cabrejo

With contributions from: Viviana Riquelme Echeverría, Consuelo Cristina Alzamora Muñoz, and Roger Rodolfo Ramírez Ramírez

Abstract

Human migratory movements, their causes, and their impacts on individuals and the larger society constitute a timely challenge for the profession. The current configuration of communities and its effects on their daily actions and occupations expose how exclusion, xenophobia, and racism, among other forms of discrimination, affect those who migrate, resulting in adverse health outcomes for migrants and the receiving communities. This necessitates occupational therapy to theoretically and practically situate, understand, and address human migration in everyday practice. Thus, this chapter intends to "re-look," interrogate, and critically reflect on the use of occupational therapy interventions based on the professional and life experience of occupational therapists who have worked with and experienced migratory processes. The authors call for co-constructing innovative occupation-based interventions relevant to the needs of subjects and territories and emphasize human rights, critical interculturality, social justice, anti-racism, and gendered approaches in occupational therapy for daily occupations that contribute to building bridges across our humanity.

Keywords

migration; critical interculturality; social justice; human rights; segregation

Learning outcomes

- Discuss how human migratory movements, and their causes, impacts, and relationships between the subjects and society, constitute a timely challenge for the profession.
- Explain the importance of occupational therapy in facilitating the social integration processes of migrants in various contexts.
- Recognize professional knowledge and practices that allow delineating the appropriate approaches in coherence with the needs of migrants in diverse contexts in Latin America and the Caribbean.

Introduction

Migration is a social phenomenon subscribed to the world of relationships, the configuration of modern societies, and the daily lives of individuals (Sassen, 2007). Although human movements are not specific to Latin America and the Caribbean, the high migratory flows and social dynamics, especially intraregional, have influenced the thoughts and actions of occupational therapists in the region. The migration of occupational therapists within and outside the region has also allowed the development and questioning of different fields of action, models of professional practice, and perspectives on human activity.

The chapter's authors and contributors have experienced migration at some point in their lives and have also worked as occupational therapists in different settings with migrant populations. Thus, they have had to learn and unlearn their daily practices, adapting to the opportunities and challenges of their contexts. From these positionalities, this chapter starts by conceptualizing migration as a plural, directly affecting the daily occupations of migrants and the receiving communities. It highlights the complexity and diversity of migratory movements and recognizes them, in the case of Latin America and the Caribbean, as byproducts of globalization and the transformations of the economic, political, social, ecological, and technological systems of the countries involved in the migration process. Furthermore, it emphasizes the need to codesign innovative occupation-based practices that respond to the occupational needs of migrant populations.

Human migration: Definition and causes

Migration is a social phenomenon with a plurality of causes, characterized by the movement of people away from their place of habitual residence, whether across an international border or within a country, regardless of:

the legal status of the migrant; the voluntary or involuntary nature of the displacement; the causes of the displacement; or the duration of their stay (IOM, 2021c), as an adaptive measure or as part of the strategies to adapt to their particular situation (Cattaneo et al., 2019).

The relevance of migration at a global level is intensified by the high rates of mobility and border crossing reported in recent years, the likelihood of increased migration in the coming decades, and the changes in migration routes and strategies. Thus, migration is a current social phenomenon affecting people's daily lives, influencing all human needs. Environmental, social, political, and economic changes will continue to make migration a common phenomenon for human survival, calling for *innovative occupational therapy practices*.

According to the International Organization for Migration (IOM), by 2020 there were 281 million international migrants worldwide (McAuliffe & Triandafyllidou, 2021), with exponential migratory growth in Latin America and the Caribbean. This plural migration comprises diverse migration groups and different causes that must be understood in a "longitudinal, long-term, multidimensional and globalising way" (Albo Díaz, 2018, p. 161). Within the parameters of international development and political visualization, as shown in Figure 7.1 the Brandt Line[1] is used to define migration patterns. These are generally described as South–North, and South–South, denoting not only the geographical area of departure and arrival but what it represents within the global social and economic system (Lees, 2021). For example, a person migrating from Argentina to Australia has a South–North migration pattern, as Australia is considered within the Global North. South–South migration examples include the recent flow from Venezuela to Colombia, Peru, and Chile.

Although there are as many reasons to migrate as there are migrants, broadly speaking there are factors at the "macro," "meso," and "micro" levels (Castelli, 2018) that, according to push and pull theory,[2] inform the decision to leave or stay (Simpson, 2017). Macro factors include economic, sociopolitical, demographic, and environmental situations. Meso factors include legal and political frameworks, the cost of migrating, technology, social networks,

1 The Brandt Line is a way of visualizing international inequalities and the socioeconomic gulf that separates regions of the world into two main economic regions: an economically powerful North and a developing South. It was first popularized in the 1980s through the *North-South: A Programme for Survival*, also known as the Brandt Report (Lees, 2021). Although the economic diversity of the South and its collective power has grown since the concept's inception, even today the Brandt Line is relevant to describe the power relations among the Global North and South nations.

2 Factors that have a push effect are the reasons why people leave a place, and those that have a pull effect are the reasons why they move to another place (Simpson, 2017).

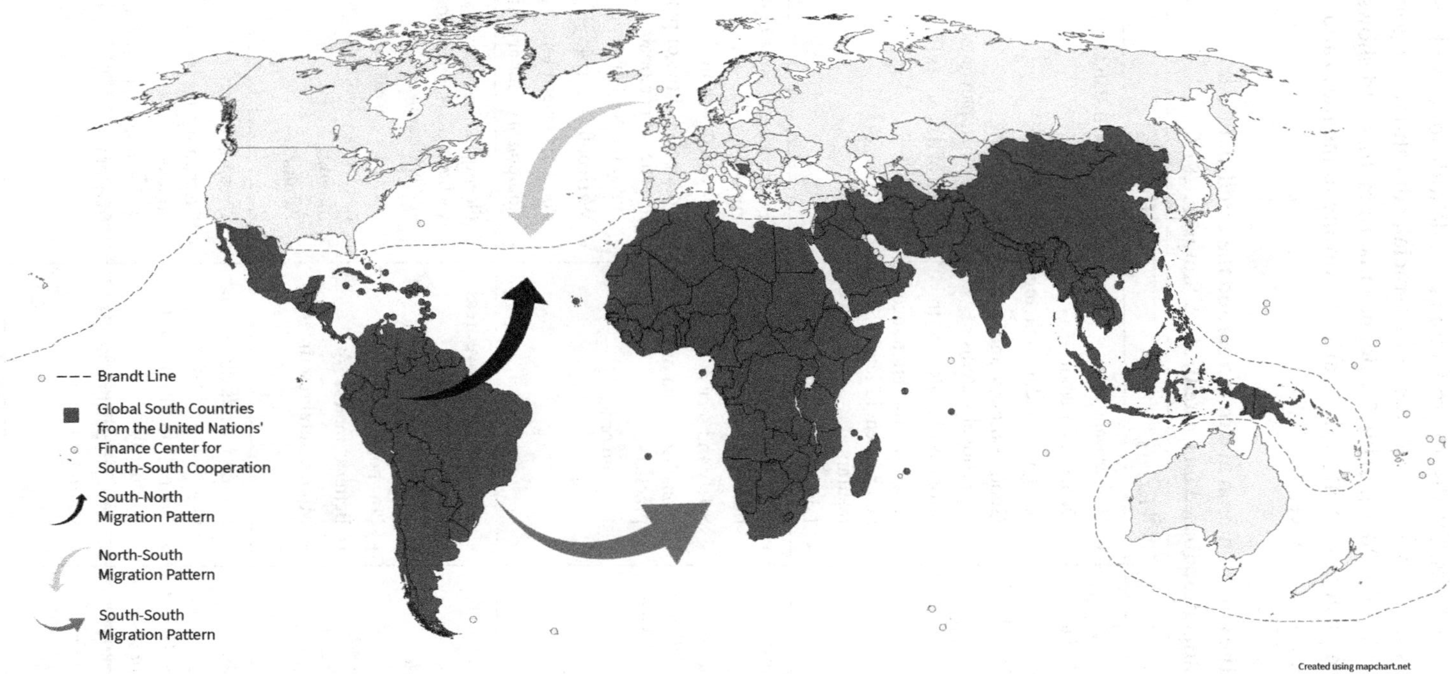

Figure 7.1 World map demarcated with the Brandt Line showing global migratory patterns (based on Lees, 2021)

and diasporic links. Finally, micro factors include individual and identity characteristics such as age, gender, ethno-racial, education, religion, and language (Castelli, 2018). Table 7.1 defines macro factors and shows how they have a push or pull effect that varies according to the meso and micro factors mentioned above.

Table 7.1 The most common macro factors and their pull and push effects on migration (based on Castelli, 2018; Simpson, 2017)

Macro factor	Pull factors	Push factors
Economic *Migration is due to labor standards, employment, and the overall health of a country's economy.*	• Higher wages • Demand for labor • A higher standard of living • Good healthcare and educational systems • Strong economic growth • Possibility for remittances and household-level insurance • Educational opportunities	• Economic instability or decline • Job insecurity • Low wages • High unemployment • Lack of incentives for higher education • High taxes
Sociopolitical *Migration is due to political and social conditions that affect one's life and views.*	• Liberal approaches to humanitarian migrants • Safety and security • Non-discriminatory practices • Law and order	• Persecution because of one's ethnicity, religion, race, politics, or culture • Country's politics or policy in issues of personal/collective need or interest • War/conflict or risk • Political persecution or risk • Compulsory military service
Environmental *Migration is due to sudden or progressive environmental changes affecting lives or living conditions.*	• Physically attractive areas of residency • Clean water • Low pollution • Better climates • More natural resources	• Fleeing natural disasters, such as floods, hurricanes, and earthquakes • Hazardous areas of residency (coasts, oil spills, mining) • Famine
Demographic *Migration is due to social networks and family ties or changes in the demographic composition that affect one's life and livelihood.*	• Family, friends, significant others, and networks • Cultural and/or linguistic familiarity • Aging population needs youth to support	• Overpopulation • Discriminatory social policies • Restriction of rights and freedoms

Research, Reflect, and Discuss

LGBTQIA+ people in El Salvador, Guatemala, and Honduras, collectively known as the Northern Triangle of Central America, face high levels of violence, have limited protections under national law, and in recent years have fled home in significant numbers, undertaking perilous journeys to seek asylum in other countries where they can be protected.

Research the current affairs for LGBTQIA+ communities in one of these countries. Consider a 20-year-old Indigenous transgender woman in the country you researched about. She is responsible for the care of her grandmother and a six-year-old nephew. After receiving multiple death threats and protecting her family from retaliation, she migrated to Mexico.

What macro factors could have been determinants for her to migrate? What pull and push factors may have taken place in her decision? How do these factors affect her daily occupations?

Contextualizing migration

As shown in Figure 7.2, when viewed in terms of international law, migration provides legal statuses that influence participation and inclusion or exclusion in everyday life. As a result, these statuses must be understood by occupational therapists—and this understanding shared with the people with whom they are working—in order to be able to codesign strategies and interventions.

Even though, in essence, the different categories are indeed migrant populations, their various legal statuses have different physical, social, emotional, psychological, and occupational implications previously documented elsewhere (Álvarez et al., 2022; Caballero et al., 2018; da Silva et al., 2020; Suleman & Whiteford, 2013; Uribe, 2017). These experiences vary according to both the departure and arrival contexts. Thus, the legal conditions in which a migrant arrives at the place of destination, or "migratory status," will significantly impact their daily life and doings. This legal status may or may not guarantee their recognition as a subject or provide acceptance and openness in the place of arrival, including access to social institutions and their services (education, health, work, citizenship, etc.). In the case where a legal status has not been granted, social descriptors of non-acceptance emerge in labels such as *irregular*, *illegal*, *undocumented*, or *unauthorized* immigrants, being unprotected and with reduced forms of action and participation (Black, 2021).

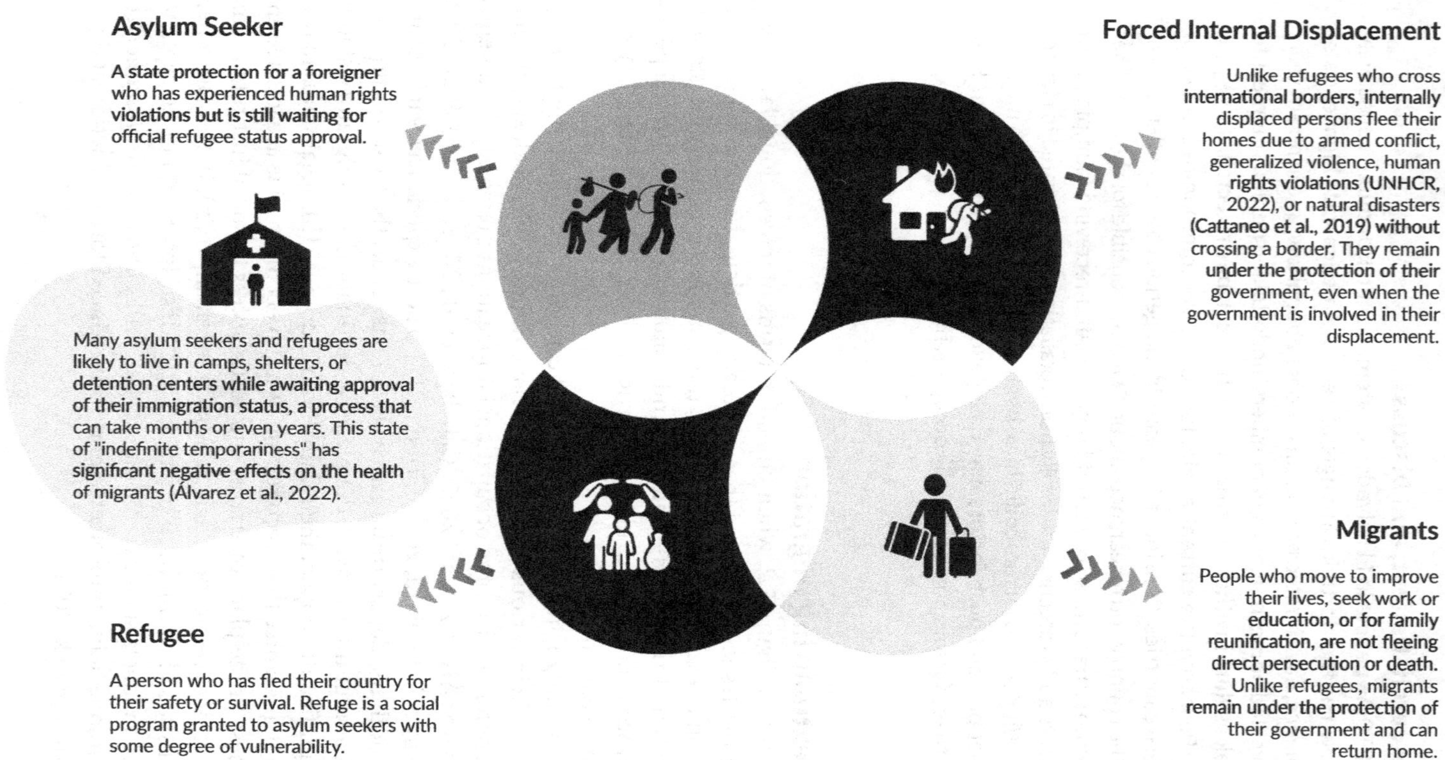

Figure 7.2 Different migration statuses (based on Álvarez, Diez, & Arberas, 2022; Cattaneo et al., 2019; UNHCR, 2022)

Many migrants lack assurances to exercise their rights as "new citizens"[3] in their arrival communities (Pulido & Veloso, 2020). It should be noted that women, children, older adults, people with disabilities, and LGBTQIA+ people are more vulnerable due to the historical exclusion to which these groups have constantly been subjected and are subject to forms of non-recognition and social contempt (Pulido, 2020). These intersectionalities[4] become crucial when it comes to an occupational therapy approach. As a result of these belittling dynamics, migrants are often perceived as a social problem, a threat, or a burden to the host society. This stigmatization reinforces hierarchical distinctions that frame "foreigners" as more desirable or legitimate than "migrants," effectively establishing a social order in which individuals are implicitly categorized as first-, second-, or third-class citizens (Sassen, 2016, 2020). These representations not only affect the individual adaptation of the migrant but also have repercussions on social and political forms of participation and inclusion in the receiving communities.

Reflect and Discuss

How has social and media representation of migrant groups affected the participation and inclusion of a social group where you live? How has that affected your daily living?

Migration flows and trends in Latin America and the Caribbean

Migration flow refers to the number of people arriving in a country (immigrants) or leaving a country (emigrants) throughout a specific period in history, depending on social changes (Polo Alvis & Serrano López, 2018). Data on these flows are essential for understanding global migration patterns and how different social and political factors in the countries of origin and destination may be related to the flow (Black, 2021). The new migration flows are transforming Latin America and the Caribbean "from a region of emigration to one of very complex movements" (Muñoz, 2021, para 4), which we will try to explain below.

3 "A new citizen is any individual who decides to migrate to a new territory, who must assume and be treated as a citizen, framed by the rights to which everyone, without distinction, has and simultaneously acquires the duties, as part of the full exercise of citizenship, participating in all social spaces like any other" (Pulido & Veloso, 2020, p. 25).

4 Defined as complex and cumulative ways of discrimination or privilege experienced by combining a person's various social and political identities.

Throughout its national and regional histories, the Latin American and Caribbean region has experienced European, African, and Asian immigration processes (Albo Díaz, 2018), emigration mainly to the United States and Europe, and more recently, intraregional South–South flows (Black, 2021).

Colonial migratory flows

Between 1492 and 1800, European empires, mainly Iberian, colonized the region, decimating Indigenous populations and trafficking enslaved people from Africa to work as forced laborers in mining and agriculture (Ferreira et al., 2018; Klein & Vinson III, 2007). The Portuguese crown prioritized the control of exports from West Africa, while the Spanish crown focused on territorial settlement in the Americas (Ferreira et al., 2018). It is estimated that between 10 and 15 million people were trafficked from the African continent across the ocean to Latin America and the Atlantic Caribbean (Klein & Vinson III, 2013). This trading system established inequitable trade relations and a social class system based on ethnoracial characteristics (see Chapter 3), with deep sociocultural wounds, such as racism and xenophobia, which still need to be healed and repaired (Rangel, 2020).

Migratory flows in the 19th century

Since the Industrial Revolution, three major patterns have emerged: foreign immigration, emigration to the United States and Europe, and intraregional migration (Albo Díaz, 2018; Pellegrino, 2003). These have been linked to environmental impacts, natural disasters, and social crises in the countries of origin (IOM, 2021a).

Foreign immigration was heavily characterized by Asian migration flows, particularly from China to Mexico, Cuba, Peru, and Brazil (Gao, 2021) and Japan to Peru and Brazil (Takenaka, 2004; Tonhati, Cavalcanti, & de Oliveira, 2022). These migrations were fueled by Japanese and Chinese government initiatives to control population growth, promote policies of industrialization and modernization of the Asian nations, and end the "problem" of impoverished peasants (Gao, 2021; Takenaka, 2004). On the other hand, they were part of the state-sponsored whitening strategies[5] across Latin America (Dos Santos, 2002).

5 State-sponsored whitening strategies are government policies that promote the assimilation of minoritized or marginalized groups into the dominant culture or population, intentionally altering racial composition based on a White imposed racial category. Across Latin America and the Caribbean, these strategies have historically included promoting European immigration, encouraging miscegenation, and propagating Eurocentric beauty standards in media and education. These policies have contributed to systemic racism and inequality in the region (Dos Santos, 2002).

Migratory flows in the 20th century

In the 20th century, the region experienced high South–North migration, primarily to the United States and Europe, driven by political, economic, and social changes during the Cold War. The two world powers at the time, the United States and the Soviet Union, attempted to impose their political model on other countries: the capitalist system versus the communist model, by establishing allied governments in Latin America and the Caribbean, giving way to dictatorial regimes, some of which are illustrated in Figure 7.3.

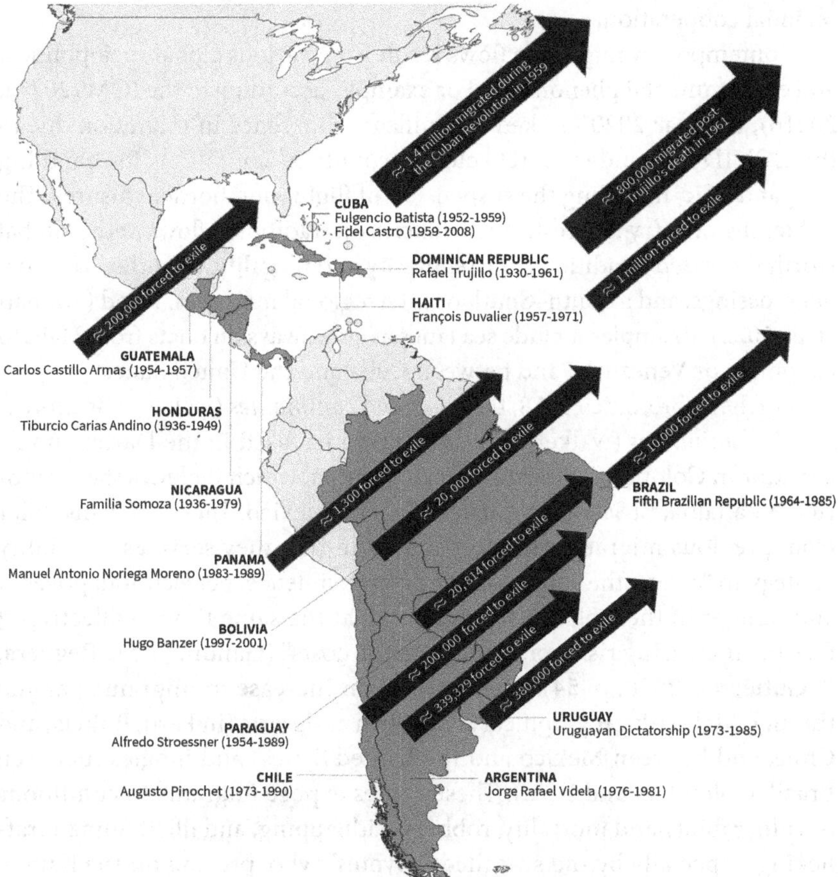

Figure 7.3 Examples of migratory flows caused by political and social changes in the 20th century in Latin America and the Caribbean (based on estimated data from CODEHUPY, 2020; Del Moral, 2020)[6]

6 For more up-to-date information about migratory flows, visit the Migration Policy Institute website at www.migrationpolicy.org

Contemporary migration flows

In general, Latin America and the Caribbean continue to receive migrants from all over the world. Such is the case of Mexico, which welcomed refugees from Afghanistan after the Taliban takeover in 2021, or Brazil, which has received a considerable number of people from Syria (Torres et al., 2022) and the Republic of Congo (da Silva et al., 2020) through their national resettlement programs and policies framed by the 1984 Cartagena Declaration on Refugees which encouraged Latin America and the Caribbean countries to make more significant provision for the protection of refugees through regional cooperation.

Contemporary migration flows result from various global sociopolitical and environmental phenomena. For example, according to the IOM (2021a, 2021b), the year 2020 marked a significant difference in migration due to the COVID-19 pandemic, reflected in countries' conditions for handling the pandemic, including the suspension of flights and border closures. The tightening of entry and restrictive policies on traditional flows to the Global North increased conditions of irregularity and illegality, unauthorized border crossings, and a South–South or interregional migration trend (Tonhati et al., 2022). Examples include sea lanes as stowaways on boats from Haiti to Colombia or Venezuela, and between Cuba and the United States.

Furthermore, since 2018, the so-called *caminantes* (walkers) or *caravanas de caminantes* (walker caravans) have increased in the Darién jungle corridor in Colombia toward Central America, which includes the territories of Panama, El Salvador, Guatemala, and Mexico. These caravans differ from previous migratory group patterns in that they serve as a mobility strategy to "escape the conditions of diverse violence, persecution, poverty, and hunger in their places of origin and, at the same time, [collectively] face the increasing risks and minimise the costs" (Gandini, de la Reguera, & Gutiérrez, 2020, p. 54). There is also an increase in migrants passing through high-risk geographical areas, such as deserts (in Peru, Bolivia, and Chile; and between Mexico and the United States) and jungles (between Brazil, Colombia, and Peru). These routes expose migrants to conditions of vulnerability and mortality, robbery, kidnapping, and illicit human trafficking, especially by the so-called "coyotes" who, preying on the human need to migrate, turn this into an illicit business that has left high rates of deaths, disappearances, and sexual violence, especially of women and children (Gandini et al., 2020).

Current migration flows have increased state control over borders, alongside efforts to protect migrants' rights. However, these flows have also intensified border defense policies and mechanisms (e.g., wall construction at the Mexico/United States border and snipers on the triple border between Bolivia, Peru, and Chile). Figure 7.4 illustrates some recent migratory routes documented by the international social research institute Instituto Tricontinental de Investigación Social (2022).

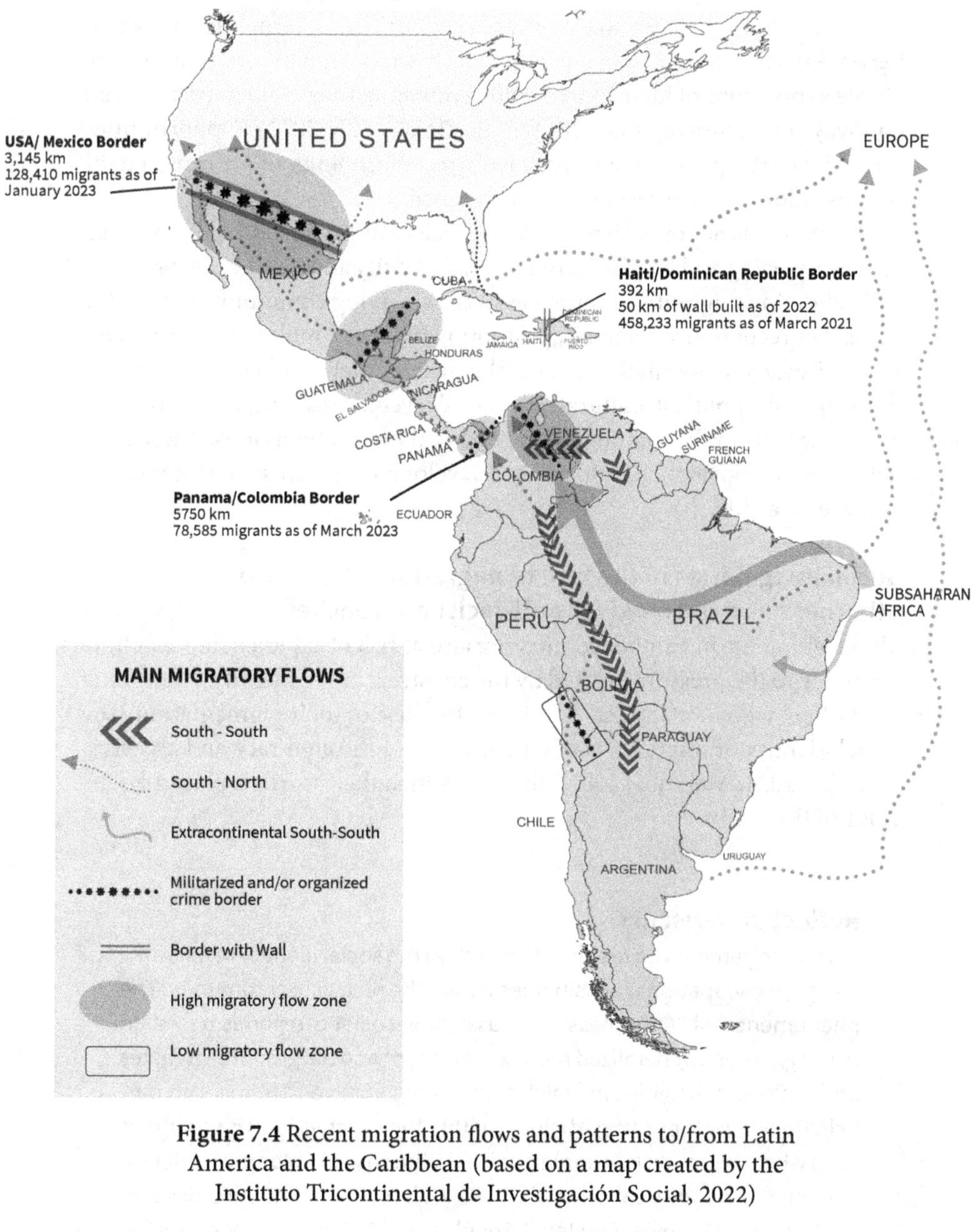

Figure 7.4 Recent migration flows and patterns to/from Latin America and the Caribbean (based on a map created by the Instituto Tricontinental de Investigación Social, 2022)

Culture, interculturality, and social identity in migratory movements

Human mobility is influenced by the social identities and culture of migrants and their host communities. Culture provides a web of collective senses and meanings that support human existence and daily activities (Talero, Kern, & Tupé, 2015). Through shared practices, humans assume identities and become part of certain social groups. In this way, human occupations are visible expressions of identity and culture, creating roles, values, preferences, and ways of occupying oneself (Trujillo Rojas et al., 2011). Opportunities for social participation in everyday living establish links and common definitions, allowing integration and coexistence.

Migration is not only about physically relocating oneself in space but also about displacing and recreating one's social identity and culture. Recognizing and validating migrants' experiences in the receiving community's everyday living can reconfigure societies, promoting diversity, multiculturalism, and interculturalism (Kymlicka, 2001). The development and contributions at the economic, political, cultural, and social levels are essential contributions of migrants from the moment of their arrival in new territories. These contributions are born, materialized, and developed in microsocial interaction and everyday life.

Social imaginaries in the face of migration: The case of otherness and the need for anti-racist approaches

Those who settle in another country are also at risk of experiencing acculturation due to the pressure exerted by the construction of identity concerning an "Other" who is attributed inferiority because of their pigmentation. The social identity of migrants is often constructed through race and colorism (Charles, 2021; Mbembe, 2006), through which their worth is placed on the color of their skin.

Reflect and Discuss

Social assignments have a direct impact on the social identity of migrants and their occupational possibilities within the receiving community. The phenomenon of "Otherness" (i.e., assigning social categories based on stereotypes and generalized representations of a social group) segregates and limits the activities in which those categorized as "Other" can participate or how they can participate within those activities. This happens even when migration is intraregional, as in the case of Colombian migrant women (Fernández Labbé et al., 2020; Pulido, 2020) and Afro-descendent women (Segovia, Aguilar, & Sepúlveda, 2018) in Chile; Venezuelan migrants in Colombia (Carrillo, Contreras, & Carreño, 2019); and Haitian migrants in Brazil (Ruiz, Robles, & Pino-Morán, 2021), among others. Intraregional migration is not exclusive to Latin America, but a rather common phenomenon around the world.

Research one of the groups mentioned above or another migratory group you are aware of in your region. How do their social labeling and representations make them feel like the "Other"? How does this "Othering" affect their daily living and the everyday living of people that look like them? How can an anti-racist approach improve occupational possibilities and participation?

These first configurations give way to social and occupational segregations that have a historical base in the colonial-modern history of the region. Thus, the organization of human groups with Western aspirations was built on the idea that the White race was at the racial summit (Charles, 2021; Mbembe, 2006). Their phenotype was related to their supposedly privileged morality and functioned as a comparative model to which other social groups aspired to approach. Part of these forms of forced rapprochement is the practice of whitening (from crossbreeding to the application of products to achieve whiteness), which persist in the region today.

Racism as a social, cultural, and political phenomenon represents a large part of the current social behavior that occurs at structural, institutional, and personal levels due to the organization of modern capitalist societies (Mbembe, 2006). For those who migrate within the region, this structural racism is combined with other identity assignments of gender, class, and socioeconomic status that determine their social mobility within the receiving community positively or negatively. Therefore, understanding the intersectionality of gender, age, place of origin, sexual identity, and economic status is vital to accompanying the forms of occupational participation of migrants and their possibilities of integration into the community (Magliano, 2015; Vigoya, 2016).

Occupational changes and migration

Mobilizations, whatever their nature, will inevitably affect the capacity of individuals to participate in individual or family roles, routines, and habits, generating a process of constant physical, mental, and emotional construction and deconstruction. On the one hand, they generate possibilities and opportunities for action and life transformation, but also tensions and challenging and stressful situations (Achotegui, 2012).

When the decision to migrate is forced under extreme conditions, leaving behind or abandoning what has been built up and familiar, added to a traumatic journey, can involve mourning processes, known as migratory mourning or Ulysses syndrome. This mourning refers to a complex process of reorganization of the personality that human beings must face to adapt to migratory change (Achotegui, 2012). These processes can affect people's ability to participate, return to a sense of occupational balance, adapt, and take on new roles, routines, and habits (Achotegui, 2012).

The transformations of daily life are usually possible through interdisciplinary collaboration, directing and managing support networks, and accompanying therapeutic processes that account for coordinated actions and a comprehensive intersectional approach to care. This is vital, especially when migrants do not know the local language and have not had previous contact with the local culture, objects, or services (e.g., how to use an electric cooker or public transportation, or how to navigate different types of employment, such as formal jobs, gig work, or self-employment). Many refugees in shelters and camps or during resettlement processes experience these issues with profound changes in individual and collective doing and being (Álvarez et al., 2022; Suleman & Whiteford, 2013).

Migration modifies dimensions that condition participation in occupations, leading to reorganizing social identities and redimensioning of occupation. Migrants must cope with new spaces, new technologies (electric cookers, alarms, heating systems, etc.), new identities, and new relationships (e.g., children who speak the language and advocate for their parents' needs). Remunerated activities are a priority in most adaptation processes, as the livelihood of the migrant and their family depends on it, even in cases where the family continues to reside in another country (i.e., sending remittances) (Omanović & Langsley, 2023). The success of this transformation depends on the host country's access and protection policies and the community's support for inclusion.

Migrants often take on new and unfamiliar occupations to adapt to the new culture, often associated with working life, which is not always pleasant or meaningful (Suleman & Whiteford, 2013). For example, due to socioeconomic conditions in Latin America and the Caribbean, many migrants are motivated to improve their families' income, often resorting to unskilled work, hazardous labor, or unsafe working conditions in their receiving communities. These changes in occupation reconfigure and, in many instances, eliminate other occupational forms related to enjoyment (e.g., play, recreation, leisure) or participation and political and civic activities (voting, electing representatives, belonging to trade union organizations or political parties, denouncing abuses, etc.).

Additionally, community occupations can be affected by a lack of social networks and limited access to services, leading to emergent occupations that play an essential role in reformulating a person's identity. Therefore, understanding both factors influencing migration and occupations from the migrant's everyday life is essential for assisting integration as an occupational therapist.

Occupational therapy and migration

Latin American and Caribbean histories of constant movement have led the profession to understand occupation as a subjective, sociocultural, and ecological process, a praxis in permanent transformation (Trujillo Rojas et al., 2011). This is important because the construction of knowledge about occupation influences occupational therapy practices (Martín & Miralles, 2013). The invitation is to consider migration as a continuous change of occupation so that, as occupational therapists, we accompany the process of those who migrate from different spaces of everyday life, including shelters, camps, schools, health centers, and community programs.

In this way, intervention devices[7] for migrants must have characteristics such as *interdisciplinarity*[8] and *transdisciplinarity*,[9] generating actions and resolving social problems. While occupational therapy is essential in the processes of adaptation, integration, and transformation through everyday activities, collaborative work with other disciplines allows us to address the variety of nuances that play a role in the participation and inclusion of migrants in the daily life of the communities where they arrive. It is proposed then that interdisciplinary and transdisciplinary actions, from an occupational perspective, should aim at social accompaniment and codesign under critical interculturality, anti-racist practices, a human-rights approach, the pursuit of social justice in everyday practices, and a gender approach, as explained below.

7 A set of actions and strategies designed to enhance people's social conditions across various spheres and contexts. Social intervention mechanisms are implemented at specific times, tailored to individuals and their recognized needs. These interventions yield better outcomes by fostering coordination among public and private social institutions, state policies, and community networks that support individuals and their environments.

8 Refers to integrating knowledge and methods from different disciplines, using a real synthesis of approaches.

9 Refers to creating a unity of intellectual frameworks beyond the disciplinary perspective.

Social accompaniment and codesign of occupational transformations

The accompaniment of migrant populations involves considering the affective aspects of human relationships, establishing therapeutic relationships, and interacting with their daily life and context. This accompaniment is based on attentive listening to the demands of individuals, groups, or collectives, often determined by vulnerability, social inequality, and lack of access to social services and essential goods (Esquerdo et al., 2015).

Therefore, occupational therapists working with migrant populations must consider three aspects of accompaniment:

- distance (where they are coming from)
- temporality (when and under what circumstances they move)
- intentionality (why they move).

These aspects are linked to people's occupational processes and suggest different accompaniments, addressing stress responses in interaction with others through strategies for empowerment and strengthening resilience.

For example, in a border shelter in Ciudad Juárez, a self-sustaining interdisciplinary program including occupational therapy allows migrants to engage in roles and routines through growing vegetables and raising farm animals, activities familiar to those who migrate to this area (Martínez Almanza & Márquez Melchor, 2022). This experience nurtures a connection with the local territory from an ecosocial perspective (Ung et al., 2020).

Another example is an interdisciplinary program in Chile's cities Temuco and Santiago that uses a gender care perspective for managing, collecting, and delivering basic groceries for Haitian and Venezuelan migrant women. It aims to balance the social gaps evidenced during the pandemic and maintain occupations related to the purchase and preparation of food, care for others and their families, and community food management for community potlucks. These community activities allow bounding and exchanging knowledge to create other projects (e.g., celebrating festivities specific to migrant communities, support networks, productive projects, training days). These daily actions allow the codesign from the experience of those who migrate with actions relevant to their context and occupational processes.

Consciousness from the Narrative in the New Way of Being and the Individual and Collective Doing to Become: The Experience of New Citizens

New Citizens is "an intercultural collective organised by migrants who have decided to become Chilean citizens and who offer help to other migrants in maintaining their cultural identity and, at the same time, their incorporation into Chilean society" (Pulido & Veloso, 2020, p. 21). This experience emerged in the Araucanía, in Temuco, Chile, and offers a space for networking and narratives, providing immediate support for basic needs such as: shelter and food through a community wardrobe; social and spiritual support through weekly meetings focused on addressing migratory mourning and elaborating life projects; and professional training on issues related to new citizenship and migration through workshops with participatory methodologies and networking (Pulido & Veloso, 2020).

Even though this is not specifically an occupational therapy program, it can illustrate how intervention through occupation takes place in interdisciplinarity, from meaningful action the expression of *ser y estar*,[10] and the social fabric is built. At the same time, the process also reveals the importance of claiming human rights, navigating systemic exclusion, and creating a roadmap for settling into and shaping the new territory they now inhabit.

Reflection question

How can we develop possibilities for codesigning empowerment and resilience-building strategies with migrants from occupational therapy accompaniment in different practice settings in the Global North?

Supportive approaches

Critical interculturality

Critical interculturality is defined as a process, project, and strategy that attempts to build radically different relationships—of knowing, being, power, and life itself (Walsh, 2009). Critical interculturality in interventions with migrants allows for articulating occupational therapy in the migrants' environment and daily life (doings). It also implements different forms of intervention between the family and social institutions by activating and managing networks (Pulido, 2022).

10 See footnote 14 in Chapter 4.

Critical intercultural approaches involve considering the migrant and their country of arrival's cultural aspects, resulting in new forms of social interaction and interculturality (Pulido & Veloso, 2020). This leads to new practices and ways of living together, fostering a sense of belonging and relating to the living space. For example, occupational therapists can participate in placemaking,[11] where migrants and communities create public spaces for exchange, restoration, and healing, such as making murals, festivals, and educational events, fostering dialogue, and imagining social possibilities (Johansson et al., 2013).

Migrant movements contribute significantly to economic, political, cultural, urban, and architectural development in the new territories of arrival. These contributions are born and developed through microsocial interactions and everyday life, forming relationships between migrants and local inhabitants. Thus, social participation, the creation of social ties, multicultural citizenship, and social recognition are fundamental for migrant integration, inclusion, and intercultural processes (Kymlicka, 2001; Tubino, 2005; Walsh, 2009).

Migrants create spaces for equity and social participation while achieving cultural assimilation and integration through learning in their new context. This transition leads to *new citizenship*, understood as their personal and social configuration in everyday life that enables full social participation. In this manner, interculturality involves complex cultural relations, negotiations, and exchanges between people with different knowledge, practices, and principles. This interaction acknowledges the "social, economic, political, and power asymmetries and institutional conditions that limit the possibility of the 'other' being considered a subject with identity, difference, and agency—with the capacity to act" (Pulido & Veloso, 2020, p. 32).

One of the effects of globalization on the integration of knowledge and practices is that it promotes exchange and diverse cultural experiences in a lively way. In the same process, social groups incorporate these affluents in various ways, broadening the possibilities for intercultural exchanges. The profession is living proof of these effects (Leiva, 2018), and its development undoubtedly depends on engaging in critical intercultural dialogues such as those proposed in this book.

Human rights approach

Human rights are an interdisciplinary and transdisciplinary approach to work, providing an ethical, moral, legal, and protective reference for societal

11 Placemaking is a philosophy and an iterative, collaborative, community-led process for creating public spaces with shared value.

coexistence. They guide protection mechanisms, such as general treaties and international covenants, that socially recognize migrants and their rights as human beings regardless of their legal status at the place of arrival (e.g., UN Convention on the Elimination of All Forms of Racial Discrimination 1965, UN Convention on the Elimination of All Forms of Discrimination Against Women 1979, UN Convention on the Rights of the Child 1989, and UN International Convention on the Protection of the Rights of All Migrant Workers and Members of Their Families 1990).

These protection mechanisms are crucial in social intervention plans and strategies, promoting dialogue and action among private and public institutions, receiving communities, and migrants. However, their effectiveness depends on countries ratifying and implementing them through laws. Therefore, occupational therapists need to familiarize themselves with these mechanisms and contribute to designing care teams as professionals, citizens, and agents of change, using critical analysis to address oppression and the subjugation of human freedom, even if individuals choose to conform, resist, or navigate these structures in different ways (Guajardo Córdoba & Galheigo, 2015). The human-rights platform can then be used to improve intercultural processes from both individual and collective levels in interventions.

Anti-racist practices

As previously discussed, migrants are often racialized in their territories of arrival based on social representations, often marked by stereotypes and racism. These representations dehumanize migrants and make their presence invisible, such as in the case of invisible jobs or activities, also known as "invisible economies of care" (e.g., personal carers, farm workers, miners, "back of the house" of a restaurant or hotel, construction workers). These daily occupations can be a double-edged sword, allowing them to participate in the community but also controlling and discriminating how they participate, facilitating their exploitation (Báez, 2022).

Recognizing migrants as citizens and agents of change provides opportunities for occupational therapists to facilitate access to everyday life. However, occupational therapists must practice critical reflexivity before intervening, recognizing the inconsistencies between their thoughts and actions, the activities to which they have (and do not have) access within the community, and the explicit and implication conditions for their participation (Talero et al., 2015). Thus, accompanying migrants' daily occupations in the host community are crucial for codesigning actions for social transformation and recognizing migrants within the communities of arrival. To effectively do this, occupational therapists must intentionally address biases, monitor roles, and unlearn racist and ableist practices. Critical self-reflection, continuous learning, and dialogue are crucial for creating inclusive and equitable environments where migrants flourish.

Social justice

Social justice is a moral and epistemic framework for occupational therapy practice (Pulido, 2022). Social justice has been a central focus in practice because of the social, economic, and political transitions experienced in Latin America and the Caribbean. It refers to the common good and *Buen Vivir* (good living, as discussed in Chapter 2), emphasizing collective care and community involvement as a primary strategy for a dignified and fulfilled life.

Occupational therapy aims to improve living conditions and opportunities for participation at various social levels, recognizing plurality, difference, and reciprocity among social actors, including occupational therapists. As an approach to practice, social justice aims to create bridges between migrant and their society of arrival, promoting social development with equal conditions, recognition, and redistribution, ultimately achieving social justice.

Case Study

Jean is a 17-year-old Haitian teenager who lived for five years in Santo Domingo, Dominican Republic, after migrating from Port-au-Prince, Haiti. In 2022, he migrated to Chile with his younger sisters (aged 15 and 12). Jean reunited with his mother, who had been living in Santiago, Chile, for a year and a half. Jean's mother had formed a family in Chile with a Haitian man with five-year-old twins. They all share a light-material house in the commune of Renca with limited access to basic services and the internet. There is only one bedroom, so the younger children sleep in shared beds.

Jean had to repeat his last year of study in a public school in Chile, which allowed him to have his first educational experience in a popular commune in Santiago (Conchalí). There he felt the pressure to adapt quickly to relationships with Chilean teenagers and other nationalities he did not know, such as teenagers from Peru and Bolivia. The family situation forced Jean to care for his younger siblings, as the adults had to spend most of their time in paid work. For this reason, Jean had to put his school and leisure activities, among other things, on the back burner. He also had to sell goods on the street to support his mother.

The family environment was very tense, mainly because of the parenting style of the stepfather, who was very restrictive and controlling toward all family members. This was exacerbated by economic, psychological, and physical violence, mainly directed at Jean.

Migra Mujer is a community support space that offers occupational therapy services in a community space where individual accompaniment and group participation are offered, especially for women who have migrated and their children. Jean comes to participate individually, which allows for a definition of objectives focused on his needs, interests, values, and age, among others. Jean wants to build spaces for leisure and free time.

How can you help Jean to build such spaces from critical interculturality and human-rights perspectives/approaches? What aspects should you consider for Jean to participate in leisure activities in his new community?

Gender focus

Gender perspectives and feminisms contribute to the denaturalization of power dynamics and domination that hinder women and girls who have migrated from accessing equality and dignity. A gender perspective in social interventions allows for contextualized and situated interventions and ensures the real protection of women's rights, particularly migrant women (Spigno, 2021).

Migration often leads to discrimination and social non-recognition for women, who are judged based on "neglect," "unprotectedness," and "abandonment" when deciding to migrate. This emotional burden increases vulnerability to mistreatment and exploitation in their arrival places as migrant women are often employed in the invisible jobs previously discussed and have historically assumed care roles for their families. As Báez (2022) explains, global care chains are constantly dominated by women, where aspects of inequality and discrimination against migrant women are evident.

Latin American countries have typically adopted *gender-sensitive* policies for irregular or undocumented migrant women, ensuring their right to sexual and reproductive health. Argentina, Mexico, and Peru have established the right to access to health services in their immigration laws, while Bolivia and Guatemala specify access to women's sexual and reproductive health services (Spigno, 2021). Occupational therapy is crucial in addressing these issues in everyday life at the individual level through direct intervention and at the population level through public policymaking.

Why a Gender Approach?

According to data from the IOM (2021a), 52.1% of international migrants are currently men, and 48% are women, a proportionally equal number. However, even though this phenomenon is not new, in recent times the invisibility of female migrants has become evident, presenting migration factors and dynamics around men (Torrado, 2014). This is relevant, as the gender aspects of such an important phenomenon as migration are ignored (Spigno, 2021). Migration due to globalization tends to feminization. This pattern increases the statistics and the social composition, trajectories, and specific vulnerabilities of migrant women (Camacho Solís, 2013; Guizardi, Gonzálvez, & Stefoni, 2018; Mora, 2008; Pulido & Muñoz, 2022).

Women's participation has specificities and deep meanings associated with global economic transformations, the restructuring of labor markets, and the consolidation of social and family networks. This also has the potential to open up more spaces for women while at the same time threatening to perpetuate patterns of gender inequality and the reproduction of the sexual division of labor associated with domestic and care work (Martínez & García, 2018; Pulido & Muñoz, 2022).

For example, caring for the home, child-rearing, and caring for any family member requiring special care assumes the naturalization of gender roles. Although the conditions of women in mobility are becoming more complex, they are still required to carry them out, with implications such as wear and tear, overload, and adverse effects on their health, as well as not having time to carry out other activities that would allow them, for example, to advance in their professional development and have better conditions for finding work.

Reflection questions

Choose a specific social group (e.g., children with disabilities, single mothers, transgender men, informal caregivers, etc.). Investigate what health services are essential for them as migrants in the country/town where you live. What policies and resources are available to them? How does access to these resources affect their daily living? Why is a gendered approach needed or not in occupational therapy? Discuss with your class.

Migrant occupational therapists

As mentioned at the beginning of this chapter, the authors and contributors are migrants. As such, they have had to redefine their everyday doings. These experiences have taught them to be sensitive to the social and occupational aspects of individual and collective migration processes and their practices in different contexts.

These occupational therapists' practices have evolved due to legal validation (i.e., validating their professional titles) and social systems (i.e., what an occupational therapist can or cannot do, and the procedures to comply with local regulations). This recognition process is often challenging, prompting authors to reflect critically, theoretically, and experientially on their personal and professional roles and actions in migratory contexts.

The authors acknowledge their social positions in diverse global contexts, including ethnicity, skin color, gender, and social class. They also recognize their privilege as practitioners and occupational therapy professors in Latin America and further afield. Thus, this chapter rescues epistemic and other essential aspects of their interdisciplinary dialogues about best addressing relevant and evolving social phenomena, such as migration, by rethinking and positioning the profession in these contexts.

Migrant or Foreigner? The Experience of a Migrant Occupational Therapist in Haiti

Migrating to Haiti has been an experience full of learning, both professionally and personally. Although this is my third experience living outside of Chile, Haiti is where I have lived the longest after Chile (11 years), allowing me to experience different situations and experiences as a migrant. I decided to live in Haiti due to my convictions and motivations, not a forced migration as many others experience on our continent. However, we often have similar experiences due to not being in our own country and facing a new culture.

Although Haiti is on our continent, its culture and language differ greatly from the rest of Latin America. It is worth remembering that Haitian culture is a mixture of European (French and Spanish) and African traditions, its official languages are French and Creole, and most of the population is Black and of African-descent.

I am the "blan" (the White one) in Haiti. I remember at first being annoyed because children would shout it at me in the street. My patients made no effort to learn my name. They would say, "Hey, blan." When I went to the market, they would charge me double because of my skin tone. It's not easy to be the "different one." Sometimes I have been advised to stay home as it can be dangerous to be on the streets, especially when the country is going through sociopolitical crises. Sometimes, I have suffered insults and threats from some people who, without even knowing what country I come from, have had an aggressive attitude. The color of my skin reminds them of the countries that have subjugated and oppressed them throughout their history. However, most of the time here, I am seen as the "foreigner," the "expatriate," but never as the migrant. Generally, people do not migrate to Haiti; however, Haitians migrate to other countries. This "status" sometimes grants privileges, which are often uncomfortable, just for having a different skin color.

Entering another culture is not easy. There must be an adaptation and transformation of both parties, the one who arrives and the one who receives. Also, migration experiences are unique, each story is different, and each person has a unique relationship with the country, the culture, and the people. I believe that individual personal factors are one of the most critical aspects in this process, which are defined by personal histories, values, tastes, adaptability, flexibility, and resilience that one can have in the face of diverse situations in a place that is not one's own.

My experience as a migrant has been primarily positive, mainly because I have had the opportunity to continue exercising my role as an occupational therapist and to develop myself in the professional field by carrying out various projects that have allowed me to feel personally fulfilled. In addition, I have integrated into my community by creating social ties with different people and actors. Although this has been a prolonged process of learning and unlearning, it has been worth it; and, despite all the problems in this country today, Haiti has become my home, where I belong now.

Conclusions

- Integrating cultural competencies into the intervention process is crucial for effectively caring for migrants in any context. Sensitivity and attention to cultural issues are essential components of practice.
- From the initial meetings, professionals should explore social and cultural identity aspects to define intervention strategies and explicitly incorporate them into the process.
- Occupation-based interventions can provide a respectful and safe space for intercultural encounters. These interventions should not

necessarily adhere to hierarchical structures dictated by the institutional context.

- Postgraduate training and specialization in interdisciplinary subjects such as legal and human rights, social welfare, public policy, management, and governance are always necessary.
- Interventions for migrant women, refugees, individuals with irregular "status," and minors require a gender perspective, considerations of human rights, protection against smuggling and trafficking, and a focus on social justice. Additionally, corporeality and interculturality should be addressed when coexisting with individuals from different backgrounds.
- Constructing social and community networks should be guided through various platforms, including health education and community-based initiatives.
- Power dynamics in healthcare settings often prioritize professional opinions, making it challenging to establish alternative modes of interaction. However, occupational therapists can contribute to creating safe spaces that facilitate individuals' transition back into the community.
- Shared occupations mediate knowledge exchange, identity formation, and cultural learning.
- Experiences with migrants from Latin America and the Caribbean highlight the importance of interdisciplinary and inter-institutional collaboration to develop integration and intercultural policies, provide orientation, support services, and foster social networks.
- Daily interactions between migrants and non-migrants shape relationships at different levels. Social participation, the formation of social ties, multicultural citizenship, and social recognition are vital for assimilation, integration, and intercultural processes (Kymlicka, 1995; Tubino, 2005; Walsh, 2009).

References

Achotegui, J. (2012). Emigrating today in extreme situations: The Ulysses syndrome. *Aloma: Revista de Psicologia, Ciències de l'Educació i de l'Esport, 30*(2), 79–86.

Albo Díaz, A. N. (2018). Being and looking Latino in the United States and Europe: Analysis of globalized perceptions. *Revista Novedades en Población, 14*(28), 160–167.

Álvarez, N. M., Díez, E., & Arberas, E. J. (2022). Analysis of functioning and participation in activities of daily living in Sahrawi refugee camps. *Journal of Occupational Science, 29*(2), XXIII–XXXV. https://doi.org/10.1080/14427591.2022.2044445

Báez, M. F. A. (2022). Migration, inequality and labor segregation: A prelude to global care crises. *Revista sobre Estudios e Investigaciones del Saber Académico,* (17), e2023001. https://doi.org/10.70833/rseisa17item339

Black, J. (2021). *Global Migration Indicators 2021*. Geneva: International Organization for Migration.

Caballero, A., Moreno, A. F., Ruíz, S. G., Navas, A., & Moreno-Sosa, M. (2018). Occupational therapy and forced human displacement, Colombia, February 2012. *Revista Ocupación Humana, 18*(1), 65–70.

Camacho Solís, J. I. (2013). The rights of migrant workers. *Revista Latinoamericana de Derecho Social,* (17), 197–258.

Carrillo, W. M. R., Contreras, A. E. T., & Carreño, F. R. D. (2019). Interculturality and occupational identity in Venezuelan migrants. *Care and Human Occupation, 8*(2), 16–22.

Castelli, F. (2018). Drivers of migration: Why do people move? *Journal of Travel Medicine, 25*(1). https://doi.org/10.1093/jtm/tay040

Cattaneo, C., Beine, M., Fröhlich, C. J., Kniveton, D., et al. (2019). Human migration in the era of climate change. *Review of Environmental Economics and Policy, 13*(2), 189–206.

Charles, J. (2021). Colorism and the Afro-Latinx experience: A review of the literature. *Hispanic Journal of Behavioral Sciences, 43*(1–2), 8–31.

CODEHUPY. (2020). *Open Windows: Report of the Truth and Justice Commission on the Dictatorship in Paraguay 1954–1989.* Coordinadora de Derechos Humanos del Paraguay.

da Silva, A. M. B. F., de Figueiredo, N. M. A., da Silva, A. B. F., da Silva, O. L. R., et al. (2020). A afetividade e acolhimento como ferramenta de inclusão na educação de refugiados. *Brazilian Journal of Development, 6*(4), 18366–18376.

Del Moral, M. (2020). Los éxodos de la Argentina: Los momentos históricos que hicieron que muchos se hicieron que se fueron que muchos se fueron del país. infobae. www.infobae.com/sociedad/2020/09/27/los-exodos-de-la-argentina-los-momentos-historicos-que-hicieron-que-muchos-se-fueran-del-pais

Dos Santos, S. A. (2002). Historical roots of the "whitening" of Brazil. *Latin American Perspectives, 29*(1), 61–82.

Esquerdo, R., Malfitano, A. P., Silva, C. R., & Borba, P. (2015). History, concepts and proposals in Brazilian social occupational therapy. *Revista Chilena de Terapia Ocupacional, 15*(1), 73–84.

Fernández Labbé, J., Díaz Allendes, V., Aguirre Sanhueza, T., & Cortinez O'Ryan, V. (2020). Colombian women in Chile: Discourses and migratory experience from intersectionality. *Revista Colombiana de Sociología, 43*(1), 17–36.

Ferreira, R., Seijas, T., de la Fuente, A., & Andrews, G. R. (2018). The slave trade to Latin America: A historiographical assessment. In A. de la Fuente & G. R. Andrews (Eds.), *Estudios Afrolatinoamericanos: Una Introducción* (pp. 41–69). Buenos Aires: CLACSO.

Gandini, L., de la Reguera, A. F., & Gutiérrez, J. C. N. (2020). *Caravanas.* UNAM, Secretariat for Institutional Development.

Gao, J. (2021). Chinese migration to Latin America: From colonial to contemporary era. *History Compass, 19*(9), e12688. https://doi.org/10.1111/hic3.12688

Guajardo Córdoba, A., & Maria Galheigo, S. (2015). Critical reflections on human rights: Contributions from Latin American occupational therapy. *World Federation of Occupational Therapists Bulletin, 71*(2), 73–80.

Guizardi, M., Gonzálvez, H., & Stefoni, C. (2018). Of feminisms and mobilities: Critical debates on migration and gender in Latin America (1980–2018). In M. Guizardi (Ed.), *The Migration Crisis in the American Southern Cone* (pp. 53–83). New York: Springer.

Instituto Tricontinental de Investigación Social. (2022). Derribando muros: Migraciones, políticas y luchas migrantes en América. https://thetricontinental.org/es/argentina/nuestraamerica2

IOM. (2021a). Migration and migrants: Global overview. *World Migration Report 2022.* Geneva: International Organization for Migration. https://publications.iom.int/system/files/pdf/WMR-2022-ES_0.pdf

IOM. (2021b). Migration research and analysis: Recent contributions of the United Nations. *World Migration Report 2022.* Geneva: International Organization for Migration. https://publications.iom.int/system/files/pdf/WMR-2022-ES_0.pdf

IOM. (2021c). Migration and migrants: Regional characteristics and developments. *World Migration Report 2022.* Geneva: International Organization for Migration. https://publications.iom.int/system/files/pdf/WMR-2022-ES_0.pdf

Johansson, K., Laliberte Rudman, D., Mondaca, M., Park, M., et al. (2013). Moving beyond aging in place to understand migration and aging: Place making and the centrality of occupation. *Journal of Occupational Science, 20*(2), 108–119.

Klein, H. S., & Vinson III, B. (2007). *African Slavery in Latin America and the Caribbean* (2nd edn). Oxford: Oxford University Press.

Klein, H. S., & Vinson, III. B. (2013). *Historia mínima de la esclavitud en América Latina y el Caribe* [*Brief history of slavery in Latin America and the Caribbean*]. El Colegio de México.

Kymlicka, W. (1995). *Multicultural Citizenship: A Liberal Theory of Minority Rights*. Oxford: Clarendon Press.

Kymlicka, W. (2001). *Politics in the Vernacular: Nationalism, Multiculturalism, and Citizenship*. Oxford: Oxford University Press.

Lees, N. (2021). The Brandt Line after forty years: The more North–South relations change, the more they stay the same? *Review of International Studies, 47*(1), 85–106. https://doi.org/10.1017/S026021052000039X

Leiva, M. D. (2018). Occupational therapies: Migrations of knowledge and practices in Latin America. *Revista Ocupación Humana, 18*(1), 21–33. https://doi.org/10.25214/25907816.197

Magliano, M. J. (2015). Intersectionality and migrations: Potentialities and challenges. *Revista Estudos Feministas, 23*(3), 691–712.

Martín, I. Z., & Miralles, P. M. (2013). Contributions of doubly reflexive ethnography in the construction of occupational therapy from an intercultural perspective. *Revista de Antropología Iberoamericana, 8*(1), 9–48.

Martínez, M. F., & García, J. M. (2018). Migratory processes and psychosocial intervention. *Papeles del Psicólogo, 39*(2), 96–103.

Martínez Almanza, M. T., & Márquez Melchor, Y. A. (2022). El albergue San Matías de Ciudad Juárez, Chihuahua, México, una alternativa de modelo sostenible para atención a migrantes. *RIDE. Revista Iberoamericana para la Investigación y el Desarrollo Educativo, 13*(25). https://doi.org/10.23913/ride.v13i25.1372

Mbembe, A. (2006). *Necropolitics*. Luxembourg: Melusina.

McAuliffe, M., & Triandafyllidou, A. (2021). Synthesis report: Technological, geopolitical and environmental transformations shaping future migration and mobility. *World Migration Report 2022*. Geneva: International Organization for Migration. https://publications.iom.int/es/node/3506

Mora, C. (2008). Globalización, género y migraciones. *Polis: Revista Latinoamericana*, 20. https://journals.openedition.org/polis/3544#quotation

Muñoz, F. (2021, December 17). Migration in Latin America and the Caribbean: 5 keys to regional development [Blog post]. https://blogs.iadb.org/migracion/es/la-migracion-en-america-latina-y-el-caribe-5-claves-para-el-desarrollo-regional

Omanović, V., & Langley, A. (2023). Assimilation, integration or inclusion? A dialectical perspective on the organizational socialization of migrants. *Journal of Management Inquiry, 32*(1), 76–97.

Pellegrino, A. (2003). La Migración Internacional en América Latina y el Caribe: Tendencias y Perfiles de los Migrantes. CELADE. https://digitallibrary.un.org/record/498078?v=pdf

Polo Alvis, S., & Serrano López, E. (2018). The new road south: Colombian migrations to Argentina. *Papel Político, 23*(1), 131–158.

Rangel, M. (2020). Protección social y migración: El desafío de la inclusión sin racismo ni xenophobia. *Políticas Sociales*, no. 45244. Naciones Unidas Comisión Económica para América Latina y el Caribe (CEPAL). https://ideas.repec.org/p/ecr/col041/45244.html

Ruiz, L., Robles, C., & Pino-Morán, J. A. (2021). Institutionalized migrant youth: A view from the occupational therapy of the South. *Cadernos Brasileiros de Terapia Ocupacional, 29*. https://doi.org/10.1590/2526-8910.ctoAO2228

Samacá Pulido, J. (2020). Gender and migration from Honneth's philosophical perspective: Experiences of non-recognition of Colombian women workers in Temuco. In C. S. Baranda & M. Blanco-Ruiz (Eds.), *Investigación Joven con Perspectiva de Género* (pp. 88–104). Madrid: Universidad Carlos III de Madrid.

Samacá Pulido, J. (2022). Justiça social como quadro moral e normativo para intervenção social com cidadãos migrantes. *Cadernos Brasileiros de Terapia Ocupacional, 30*, e3066. www.cadernosdeterapiaocupacional.ufscar.br/index.php/cadernos/article/view/3066

Samacá Pulido, J., & Muñoz, F. (2022). Cuerpos de mujeres colombianas en Temuco, Chile: Formas (voces) de no reconocimiento y menosprecio. In C. Cirinue & F. Baltazar (Eds.), *Corpo em Foco: Proposições Contemporâneas e Cuerpo como Foco: Proposiciones Contenporáneas* (pp. 271–282). Claretiano Rede Educaçao.

Samacá Pulido, J., & Veloso, E. O. (2020). New citizens: Recognition as social justice for migrants. *Revista Interinstitucional Brasileira de Terapia Ocupacional, 4*(1), 19–26. https://doi.org/10.47222/2526-3544.rbto30526

Sassen, S. (2007). *Elementos para una Sociología de la Globalización: Una Sociología de la Globalización*. Buenos Aires: Katz Editores.

Sassen, S. (2016). Three emerging migrations: An epochal shift. *International Journal on Human Rights, 13*(23), 29–42.

Sassen, S. (2020). A new kind of migrant: Escaping "development"? *Forum: Revista Departamento de Ciencia Política*, (18), 124–144. https://doi.org/10.15446/frdcp.n18.82102

Segovia, J. S., Aguilar, F. R., & Sepúlveda, P. Z. (2018). Work experiences of Afro-Colombian migrant women in northern Chile. *Interciencia, 43*(8), 544–551.

Simpson, N. (2017). Demographic and economic determinants of migration push and pull factors drive the decision to stay or move. *IZA World of Labor*, 373. www.econstor.eu/handle/10419/171181

Spigno, I. (2021). The difficult inclusion of a gender perspective in the protection of migrant women in Latin America. *AG About Gender – International Journal of Gender Studies*, 10(20). https://doi.org/10.15167/2279-5057/AG2021.10.20.1332

Suleman, A., & Whiteford, G. E. (2013). Understanding occupational transitions in forced migration: The importance of life skills in early refugee resettlement. *Journal of Occupational Science, 20*(2), 201–210.

Takenaka, A. (2004). The Japanese in Peru: History of immigration, settlement, and racialization. *Latin American Perspectives, 31*(3), 77–98.

Talero, P., Kern, S. B., & Tupé, D. A. (2015). Culturally responsive care in occupational therapy: An entry-level educational model embedded in service-learning. *Scandinavian Journal of Occupational Therapy, 22*(2), 95–102. https://doi.org/10.3109/11038128.2014.997287

Tonhati, T., Cavalcanti, L., & de Oliveira, A. T. (2022). A decade of growth in migration in Brazil (2010–2020) and the impact of the COVID-19 pandemic. In *Migration in South America: IMISCOE Regional Reader* (pp. 99–120). New York: Springer International.

Torrado, T. L. V. (2014). El panorama migratorio internacional: Una mirada desde el género. *Sociedad y Equidad: Revista de Humanidades, Ciencias Sociales, Artes y Comunicaciones*, no. 6, 111–137. https://dialnet.unirioja.es/servlet/articulo?codigo=4846663

Torres, C. V., Safdar, S., Oliveira, S. E., Adaid-Castro, B. G., et al. (2022). Refugees in Brazil: An investigation of Syrian refugees' psychological experiences. *International Journal of Psychology, 57*(4), 466–474.

Trujillo Rojas, A., Sanabria Camacho, L., Carrizosa Ferrer, L., Parra Esquivel, E., et al. (2011). *Occupation: Meaning, Fulfillment and Freedom: Occupational Dialogues Around the Subject, Society and the Environment*. Universidad Nacional de Colombia.

Tubino, F. (2005). La interculturalidad crítica como proyecto ético-político. *Encuentro Continental de Educadores Agustinos, 1*, 24–28.

Ung, Y., Sarah, T. S., Drolet, M.-J., Simó, S., & Soubeyran, M. (2020). Building occupational therapy practice ecological based occupations and ecosystem sustainability: Exploring the concept of eco-occupation to support intergenerational occupational justice. *World Federation of Occupational Therapists Bulletin, 76*(1), 15–21.

UNHCR. (2022). Internally displaced persons. www.acnur.org/personas-desplazadas-internas.html

United Nations. (1965). *International Convention on the Elimination of All Forms of Racial Discrimination*. www.ohchr.org/en/instruments-mechanisms/instruments/international-convention-elimination-all-forms-racial

United Nations. (1979). *Convention on the Elimination of All Forms of Discrimination Against Women, New York, 18 December 1979*. www.ohchr.org/en/instruments-mechanisms/instruments/convention-elimination-all-forms-discrimination-against-women

United Nations. (1989). *Convention on the Rights of the Child.* www.ohchr.org/en/instruments-mechanisms/instruments/convention-rights-child

United Nations. (1990). *International Convention on the Protection of the Rights of All Migrant Workers and Members of Their Families.* www.ohchr.org/en/instruments-mechanisms/instruments/international-convention-protection-rights-all-migrant-workers

Uribe, J. S. R. (2017). Transculturation and its influence on activities of daily living in women victims of displacement. *TOG (A Coruña), 14*(25), 56–71.

Vigoya, M. V. (2016). Intersectionality: A situated approach to domination. *Debate Feminista, 52*, 1–17.

Walsh, C. E. (2009). *Interculturalidad, Estado, Sociedad.* Universidad Andina Simón Boliva, Ecuador: Abya-Yala.

PART 4

ARENAS

CHAPTER 8

The Neoliberal Framing of Occupational Therapy Practices and the Rise of the Health Consumer

Lisette Farias, Michelle Lapierre, and Vagner Dos Santos

Abstract

This chapter discusses neoliberalism's impact on providing occupational therapy services in Latin America. Neoliberalism is a political-economic theory and way of reasoning that promotes individualism, consumerism, competition, and meritocracy.[1] Neoliberalism permeates all areas of life, including health services, social care, and occupational therapy practices. Occupational therapists in the region hold a long commitment to democracy, justice, and participation, yet practices are embedded within neoliberal systems and commercial liberty. This false liberty is promoted as individual and professional entrepreneurial freedom within social structures such as health and social care. It is characterized by private property rights, capital accumulation and reinvestment, and free markets. This, combined with a weakening of values such as human rights, democracy, and social justice within Latin America, makes neoliberalism a robust mechanism for the continued support of the postcolonial elites that benefit from the oppression and marginalization of groups in societies. In this chapter, the authors explore the provision of occupational therapy services concerning (a) the neoliberal framing of occupational therapy practices; (b) the emergence of the health consumer; and (c) understanding occupation as neoliberal(ized),

1 Neoliberal meritocracy builds on the notion that effort and talent are enough to ensure upward social mobility, facilitating individualization and competition. This, in turn, has resulted in increasing social inequalities (Rottenberg, 2018).

situated, and colonized. These topics will be discussed and interrelated with examples from professional practices.

Keywords
neoliberalism; capitalism; healthcare provision; discourse

Learning outcomes

- Identify key features of neoliberal ways of thinking and actions related to providing occupational therapy.
- Recognize the impact of neoliberalism and capitalism on providing occupational therapy services in Latin America.
- Reflect on the importance of decolonizing occupational therapy practices to support the reclaiming of traditional occupations and knowledge.

Introduction

This chapter focuses on neoliberalism's impact on occupational therapy provision. The Latin American example is discussed to exemplify the corrosive effects of this political and economic ideology. Neoliberalism shapes social institutions, including the health system, and provides insight into the limitations and possibilities of occupational therapy practices. Although efforts have emerged (e.g., Almonacid et al., 2021; Farias & Bezerra, 2016; Prado, Silva, & Silvestrini, 2020; Reina Bolaños, 2021), the topic remains unexplored in hegemonic occupational therapy literature. On the other hand, Southern scholars have engaged and examined how neoliberalism builds from other forms of political and economic oppression. For instance, Brazilian scholars have argued for the engagement of the profession in political and economic issues such as neoliberalism and capitalism to mobilize resistance and redefine its professional relation to public and private institutions (Bezerra & Trindade, 2013; Silvestrini, Silva, & Prado, 2019). Similarly, Chilean scholars have described the influence of neoliberalism on occupational choices and its impact on people's health and well-being (Rolack Jaramillo, Triviños Rubilar, & Troncoso Henriquez, 2015) and referred to occupational therapy as a penalizing actor of the neoliberal state (Herrera Sandoval & Valderrama Nuñez, 2013).

Although these examples illustrate an increasing discussion regarding the pervasive influence of neoliberalism on social-structured problems, they also show a gap related to how neoliberalism frames occupational therapy service provision in ways that affect practitioners and the groups with whom they work. This awareness is relevant since neoliberalism promotes values and epistemology that bind professional resources and care provision (Almonacid et al., 2021; Dos Santos, 2022; Farias, 2020). Governments that promote neoliberal values such as individualism and consumerism portray individuals as capable and responsible for their health and able to choose to stay healthy (Farias, 2020). In this way, neoliberal governments promote discourses that turn health service problems into individual problems and as a matter of individual responsibility. Discourses are mechanisms of power conveyed through policies and media that promote ideal types of thinking and doing, such as what it means to be healthy, how it looks to be healthy, and what types of activities promote health (Blanchet Garneau, Browne, & Varcoe, 2019; Farias, 2020). Given the influence of neoliberalism on healthcare services and people's lives and ways of living, it is essential to shed light on how occupational therapy can prevent the reproduction of neoliberal ways of thinking and doing, and contribute to addressing structural problems that affect individuals, groups, and communities.

The authors' positionality is presented below, followed by the definition of key concepts. After this, the Latin American context is traced, followed by discussion of the impact of neoliberalism on occupational therapy and resultant professional tensions. Finally, reflections and implications for the occupational therapy profession are presented.

Positionality of the authors

This chapter's authors are committed to promoting social justice and knowledge pluralism within occupational therapy practices and using critical theoretical perspectives within our work. Lisette is a Chilean occupational therapist working as a researcher and lecturer in Sweden. Her work is within critical health research, including health professional development toward socially responsive practices and transformative education and practices. Michelle is an occupational therapist, researcher, and lecturer working in Chile. Her work includes critical disability studies, feminist theory, and intercultural studies. Vagner is an occupational therapist from Brazil working as a researcher and lecturer in Australia. Vagner's research aims to understand the production of social vulnerabilities in postcolonial realities and how occupational therapy theory and practice can address socially structured problems. His research agenda is developed at the crossroad of two fields—health and social sciences—allowing him to dialogue with a wide range of scholars and schools of thought. We are also engaged to different extents in the debate about critical/Southern occupational therapy perspectives and occupation-based social transformative theories and practices.

Our positionalities, including professional experiences, are relevant as we draw on our previous experiences as occupational therapists, research, and literature to articulate a position against the proliferation of neoliberal values in education, practice, and knowledge production. As Latinxs, we use the Latin American example to illustrate the risks of this political and economic discourse. We will also draw on critical theoretical perspectives, called critical social theory (Farias & Aldrich, 2021; Kincheloe & McLaren, 2005), to examine how neoliberal values and ideas create invisible ways to normalize social problems as things are.

Key concepts

Concepts such as *neoliberalism*, *capitalism*, and *new public management* are presented here. The first, *neoliberalism*, refers to a political-economic theory. It represents a way of reasoning that promotes a particular epistemology and practices based on values such as individualism, consumerism, competition, autonomy, and self-reliance rather than reliance on public resources (Bastías et al., 2008). Neoliberalism is also referred to in the literature as a way of thinking that promotes reducing governmental intervention in the economy, providing entrepreneurial freedoms and property rights to individuals who can compete and accumulate capital and investments. In close alliance with *capitalism*, which promotes consumerism and competition, neoliberalism promotes the idea of human flourishing as individually attainable through free market economies (Ayo, 2012). Using this reasoning, capitalist societies promote a vision of everyday life and doing shaped by what is deemed valuable, acceptable, or desirable by the free market (Esposito & Perez, 2014; Farias, 2020). Thus, the term neoliberalism is used in this chapter to denote a political-economic theory and way of governing that promotes values that follow those supported by capitalism. This, in turn, portrays personal gain or profit as morally responsible and productive forms of human agency (Esposito & Perez, 2014; Farias, 2020). It is worth noting that neoliberalism is not spread as a coherent set of ideas imposed similarly throughout the world. Instead, it is "a logic of governing that migrates and is selectively taken up in diverse political contexts" (Ong, 2007, p. 3). It manifests in different expressions, yet the values underlying neoliberal thinking and doing have become globally dominant since the 1970s (Harvey, 2007).

Although most professionals may not necessarily identify that specific neoliberal market values shape their practices and professional decisions, they might experience ethical tensions related to systemic constraints connected to broader societal disparities (Bushby et al., 2015; Durocher et al., 2016). Ethical tensions have been described in the literature related to balancing the imposed needs of healthcare system structures, resources, or policies against the needs of those we serve (Almonacid et al., 2021; Durocher et al., 2016).

Neoliberal values are often transmitted via *discourses*, which are often normalized and internalized by individuals who use them to know how to act in ways that are socially desirable or expected (Foucault, 1977). Neoliberal values become dominant through discourses that are accessible to everyone (e.g., social media, policies) and then enacted in services and everyday practices. In this way, specific neoliberal ways of thinking and practicing can be privileged over others, framing them as legitimate or universally true and defining what is desirable, ideal, or possible within a given context. Chomsky and Waterstone (2020) have discussed the implications of neoliberal discourse, or *neoliberal common sense*, in maintaining and magnifying existing inequalities.

Reflect and Discuss

What is common sense?

It is a form of "everyday thinking" that is universally true and offers a framework of meaning to make sense of the world. Experiences and personal background usually inform it. For example, an occupational therapist has been privileged with stable housing, private education, and internet access. The same occupational therapist suggests websites to clients needing information about community resources.

- What is being taken for granted by the occupational therapist in this case?
- What questions could be asked of clients before assuming their status, housing situation, and education level?

Since organizational management is a significant part of the criticism of neoliberalism, the concept of *new public management* (NPM) is also essential in this chapter. Some NPM schemes of organization and control are imported from business to public institutions, including healthcare (Molina & Tobar, 2018). Under NPM, individual workers are treated as enterprises and expected to follow a profit-making logic. This means they are held accountable to the organization through performance-management systems, so professionals must make themselves accountable in terms of competition to ensure quality or standardized results. In this way, intervention outcomes are concordant with neoliberal measures (e.g., austerity), pressuring professionals such as occupational therapists to achieve cost-effectiveness and accountability by promoting such strategies as simplification, categorization, and reductionism. These strategies are problematic since they impose limits and restrict possibilities for developing socially responsive practices by making other factors invisible or irrelevant to managerial agendas (Farias & Rudman, 2019; Hayes et al., 2023).

Reflect and Discuss

What is neoliberal austerity?

Neoliberalism acts in ways that seek to reduce the role of the state and welfare, which pressures citizens to compete for income, wealth, and power. Since the state and welfare are reduced, austerity measures seek to reduce the state's expenditure on public services by reducing the number of professionals, programs, and healthcare services, thereby increasing the demands and unmet needs of the most vulnerable groups in society (Sakellariou & Rotarou, 2017).

- How do you think occupational therapy is affected by increasing demands for attending to more clients?
- What are the risks of introducing cost-effective mechanisms into occupational therapy practices?
- What are the implications of austerity measures for those historically neglected from services, for example Indigenous people living in remote areas?

The beginnings of neoliberalism in Latin America

Neoliberalism can be traced back to the early 1960s in Latin America, particularly in the cases of Brazil and Colombia (Fischer, 2009), and then to the 1980s and 1990s in countries such as Peru, Venezuela, and Mexico. While neoliberalism expanded its influence over the healthcare system in these countries, Chile is often described as the world's first "neoliberal" experiment. This is a unique case in which a specific form of authoritarian rule (i.e., military dictatorship[2]) paved the way for applying extensive market reforms without any opposition permitted (Rodríguez, 2021). Chile was one of the first countries to introduce neoliberal reforms in the health sector in the

2 For more information about the military dictatorship that affected Chile during 1973–1986, see Loveman (1986).

1980s, developing what is called a "free market" and an extensive marketization of its public healthcare that led to the creation and perpetuation of health inequalities in the country (Rotarou & Sakellariou, 2017). The Chilean model later influenced regional reforms pushed by international agencies (e.g., the World Bank) (Unger et al., 2008).

A *free market* is a system in which prices are determined by unrestricted competition among privately owned businesses, often ruled by local classes and corporate interests. As such, the free market is at the core of neoliberal discourse, especially in capitalist societies where individual and private profit is essential to maintain consumerism (Connell, Fawcett, & Meagher, 2009; Peacock, Bissell, & Owen, 2014). Neoliberalism often portrays the state as a deficient administrator or operating a monopoly in which entrepreneurs need to meet fixed costs and taxes and therefore promotes the de-monopolization of the market to allow private actors to find their value and set their price. Theoretically, it should be cheaper to run a de-monopolized or free market system because it is not part of the state bureaucracy and no longer part of the tax burden, "liberating" the state and consumers who can take the responsibility for choosing products based on what they can afford. As such, the free market creates an illusion that free competition guarantees quality, obscuring the fact that it also perpetuates and aggravates social inequalities between those who can and those who cannot afford products or services (Göttems & Mollo, 2020).

In general, neoliberal reforms started during the 1970s and 1980s in most Latin American countries as a developmental strategy that would support the industrialization model. However, the industrialization model was replaced instead by bureaucratic-authoritarian regimes, arising first in Brazil (1964), Argentina (1964, 1976), Chile (1973), and Uruguay (1973) under military rule (Rodríguez, 2021). The expansion of neoliberalism in the region has been described as having these common features:

- being established in countries with existing or increasing inequalities
- prohibiting and persecuting the political opposition and attacks in popular sectors either by brutal military repression or authoritarian rule
- dismantling the previous state-centric and industrial development strategy by restructuring the economy to favor the liberalization of the free market, and marketization of critical areas of social provision such as education, health, pensions, and housing
- transitioning from an industrialization model to an export-oriented model, opening up the domestic economy to the global market.

Neoliberalism was enacted differently in the region than in the Global North, where neoliberalism could coexist with a certain degree of social democratic and welfare institutions. In the Global North, although the transition to the neoliberal model involved mass unemployment and systematic confrontation with groups of workers and riots, it is considered gentle compared to the abrupt and military-controlled initiation of neoliberalism in Latin America (Rodríguez, 2021). This process established an imitation of Europe's industrialization model, which was then replaced by neoliberal reforms (and the emergence of capitalist economies) in the region. It is worth noting that the Latin American region was first subjected to European colonization—a process in which Europeans exploited the region, massacred Indigenous people, enslaved Black people, and committed epistemic genocide and mass destruction of the natural environment, which became the basis of Europe's rise in the 19th century.

Neoliberalism and its impact on occupational therapy

Neoliberal reforms introduced in Latin America since the early 1960s have led to extensive changes in the public sectors, including a severe deterioration in the quality of state healthcare services. Therefore, examining the consequences of neoliberal reforms and thinking for professions such as occupational therapy that provide services within the public and private healthcare sectors is relevant. From our view, the impact of neoliberalism on the provision of occupational therapy services in a Latin American context generates three tensions concerning:

- the neoliberal framing of occupational therapy practices
- the emergence of the health consumer and the health vendor
- the understanding of occupation as neoliberal(ized), situated, and colonized.

Neoliberal framing of occupational therapy practices

Neoliberal healthcare reforms are often presented as restructuring ineffective and costly healthcare systems by applying reductionist strategies, such as spending cuts, downsizing, and competitiveness, to satisfy the goals of the free market (Rotarou & Sakellariou, 2017). Since the 1980s in Chile, the health system has been divided into public and private to improve efficiency and lower costs. Instead, this has led to increased inequality among groups in society, mainly affecting people experiencing poverty (including the middle and working classes), older adults, and women, who are not adequately protected against ill health and its consequences.

The greatest challenge faced by the Chilean public system is the characteristics of the population it serves, which corresponds to 78% of the population, versus the private system, which attends to 14.4% of the country's population (Ministerio de Desarrollo Social [Ministry of Social Development], 2018). The population served by the public system is older, has low or no income, and has higher exposure to social determinants of health that negatively influence their health. This population needs greater resources, weakening the public system, which already receives insufficient funding for facing these challenges (Lapierre, 2020). Privatizing a large part of the services within the public system has diverted significant public funds to private for-profit companies in a system of free competition. This free competition has forced the public sector to adopt austerity measures, decreasing government budget expenditure for healthcare services, including occupational therapy, leading to salaries that cannot compete with the private system and shortages of resources. This competition can be associated with the free market promotion of job insecurity, which increases pressure to attend to as many people as possible at the expense of reducing job guarantees, union protection, and other labor rights (Rotarou & Sakellariou, 2017).

Such spending cuts also pressure professionals to compete and justify the need for one's position within private institutions (Owens, Singh, & Cribb, 2019) and create expectations for occupational therapists working in private and public sectors to work more with less support and resources. For example, budget cuts affect occupational therapists by putting their professionalism and decision-making at risk, which becomes more difficult if the practitioner is working with limited resources or in isolation since therapists are being hired for specific hours or positioned in different units/schedules. This can be unsustainable and harmful to practitioners and those they serve, causing the loss of important information, opportunities for collaboration, and provision of the same quality of care for all (Venegas Villascan & Feregrino Feregrino, 2022).

Example of How Budget Cuts Can Affect Professionalism

Professionalism is developed within a professional system and organizational context and emerges from reflexivity, ethical behavior, values, training/experience, and specific behaviors, such as working in teams, communicating properly, and advocating for people's needs (Lecours, Baril, & Drolet, 2021). However, when occupational therapists work in settings affected by budget cuts, opportunities to collaborate with interdisciplinary teams or communicate with clients and their families, particularly for post-discharge follow-up, are often reduced or eliminated from the scope of services provided (Almonacid et al., 2021).

Have you considered how changes in the organizational context affect professionalism?

The public health system in Chile suffers from deterioration in its infrastructure, inefficient management, and poor coordination between regional and municipal health services (Unger et al., 2008). As a result, practitioners risk suffering burnout and stress-related symptoms and confronting moral and ethical dilemmas in their everyday practices (Missoni & Solimano, 2010). Similarly, practitioners in the Global North have described experiencing ethical tensions related to imposed practices, ineffective processes, and a lack of services that generate broader social inequalities (e.g., Durocher et al., 2016).

On the other hand, in the private health sector, where better-quality services and timely attention are promised to those who can afford these services, there is an underlying focus on increasing profits instead of providing good-quality services. This focus on profits can increase pressure on practitioners' accountability for the cost-effectiveness of interventions, measurable outcomes, and productivity. This pressure on practitioners for the costs and quality of their services leaves very little room for professional discretion to modify interventions to fit specific client needs or situations (Farias & Rudman, 2019). Thus, neoliberalism pressures practitioners to balance demands for effectiveness versus attending to people's needs, often failing to address people's complex situations, applying biomedical reductionism to inform professional practice, and neglecting people's occupational needs (Bezerra, Lopes, & Basso, 2022).

Neoliberal strategies of reduction and effectiveness work against the flexibility required to adapt interventions to people's needs and use occupational therapists' experiential knowledge (Turcotte & Holmes, 2021). Focusing on measuring outcomes to demonstrate effectiveness works against practices that aim to be holistic or consider social processes since social complexity does not translate into standardized measures and predetermined outcomes (Sakellariou & Pollard, 2017). For example, occupational therapists working in the public health system may often encounter vulnerable populations affected by multiple health conditions and social situations (e.g., unemployment, poverty, violence). This complexity is difficult to measure and is reduced to standardized interventions or assessments that focus on individual health and neglect the social disparities in which they live (Farias & Rudman, 2019).

The emergence of the health consumer and the health vendor—health as a marketable need

A dual health system (i.e., private and/or public) within a country often results in the stratification of access to health, health inequalities, and the transformation of health services into consumer products. At the same time, the free market converts health into a marketable need rather than a human right. This transformation of health to a private good, and the loss of its regulation as a universal right, also transforms the relationship between practitioners and people (da Silva & Ferreira, 2020). Since health can be purchased, people become health consumers, and practitioners become health vendors or suppliers who must adapt to market trends to be deemed valuable or desirable. For example, some services (e.g., occupational therapy) can be framed by the private sector as more desirable than others, expecting people to pay higher prices for those products, often labeled according to societal and marketing trends.

Aligned with these trends, consumerism, or the capacity to purchase health services, becomes a status symbol. For example, being healthy depends on social capital, which also depends on being/staying healthy to maintain the social contract of transacting relationships. In the case of Chile, social and economic inequalities, along with the rise of consumerism, have reinforced a class-conscious society where being poor is synonymous with being in debt, fueling discrimination and increasing social pressure to consume as a means of social validation (Stillerman, 2012). Likewise, the body becomes a sign of physical health that reflects the capacity of an individual to consume the right products to maintain good health. This implies that health becomes a sign of power that supports the emergence of an elitist health industry (e.g., unique products and grocery stores, apps, sports clothes, and merchandise) that creates an aspirational illusion and marginalizes those who cannot afford to stay healthy (Hokowhitu, 2014). Neoliberalism in health discourse is closely aligned with ableist ideas. In this way, occupational therapy services can become more expensive and be directed only toward elites who can afford them (e.g., ergonomic counseling oriented to desk-executive jobs or rehabilitation related to sports injuries), whereas groups in most need may depend on elite fundraisings.

Neoliberalism ideology impacts the public and private sectors by promoting that individuals instead of the healthcare system are responsible for maintaining health and providing high-quality services. This emergence of individual responsibility is often framed as an opportunity for citizens to make conscious decisions about their health or take control of their health by learning self-management or self-skills (Farias, 2020). For example, privatization can place pressure on practitioners who are required to *empower* those who need the most support from healthcare services so that they are not a burden to society (e.g., having to discharge people from rehabilitation or acute settings early; having less or insufficient time to engage appropriately with people's unique conditions; having to focus on empowering as a form of ill health prevention).

Example of Elite-Funded Rehabilitation

In Chile, the largest charitable institution is Teletón, which was established under a military dictatorship as part of the health sector's structural reform, which privatized and commercialized healthcare (Húmeres, 2017). Teletón's goal was to benefit disabled people by having an annual televised fundraiser in which—following the format of its North American counterpart created by Jerry Lewis in 1966—funds are gathered for building rehabilitation centers for children in the regions where there is no or very little governmental support or public services. This configures disability as a personal medical tragedy that needs to be alleviated through the recovery of bodily focused and biomedical treatment and a paternalistic view of disabled children who depend on the elite for financing their rehabilitation (Húmeres, 2017).

Have you considered how charitable and governmental institutions portray disability and how this image hinders or facilitates the social participation of people with disabilities?

The Problem of Empowerment

Empowerment has been defined in occupational therapy literature as the process of transforming "visible and invisible relationships so that power is shared more equally" (Hammell, 2016, p. 282). However, its application has been criticized since there has been little or no effort among professionals to engage in issues of power, either in the relationships between therapists and clients or within the social contexts of which they are both part (Hammell, 2016). Empowerment has been associated with enabling, which can be interpreted as occupational therapists having the power to allow opportunities and give abilities or voice to people (who then are seen as powerless) and placing occupational therapists as experts (perpetuating unequal power relations). Using empowerment as a core concept can also risk thinking that the power to change situations resides within the individual who is too lazy, irresponsible, or not a good citizen to change their lifestyle. For instance, occupational therapists working from an empowerment approach can (un)consciously focus on what people do or feel about what they do to change their lives, assuming that the responsibility is on the individual while overlooking contextual social factors, such as marginalization and poverty.

Have you considered using empowerment concerning power among clients and therapists?

Problematizing the discourses of health consumers and individual responsibility for maintaining health has been described (e.g., Farias & Rudman, 2019; Rudman, 2013) concerning the profession's long relationship with a biomedical perspective. This biomedical, able-body, or body-focused training benefits from neoliberal values by reducing disease resulting from human action and health as a product of individual enterprise (Farias, 2020; Navarro, 2008; Rose, 2013). Pérez (2021) argues that "it is highly likely that we are functionally contributing to capitalism without realizing it in the educational processes in occupational therapy" (p. 1545). This implies that with neoliberal values in university education, students are being trained as entrepreneurs who can use their skills in a marketplace through which profits can be made, perpetuating the circle of consumption of rehabilitation services (Dos Santos, 2022; Pérez, 2021).

Understanding occupation as neoliberal(ized), situated, and colonized

Questioning neoliberal principles in occupational therapy is possible and necessary (Dos Santos, 2022). To advance this intent, the contributions made to the profession by some philosophies and critical social theory (i.e., critical theoretical approaches), such as feminism, environmentalism, interculturality, and decoloniality, are significant. These approaches have nurtured proposals such as feminist occupational therapy, occupational therapies from the South, and ecosocial occupational therapy (e.g., Grandón Valenzuela, 2019; Lopes & de Oliveira, 2022; Pizarro et al., 2018; Valderrama Núñez, Sepúlveda Hernández, & Hermosilla Alarcón, 2021).

One of the profession's most significant challenges is to move beyond the notion that critical perspectives are not exclusively meant to be used in the community or social occupational therapy (Irvine-Brown, Ware, & Malfitano, 2022; also see Chapter 9 of this book). On the contrary, they are essential and useful in all scenarios where the profession is enacted, including clinical ones where the dominant biomedical model prevails. No person or institution exists independent of social and political contexts. This notion is fundamental in the practices where the person is still seen as separate from sociocultural and political influences.

Latin America is facing challenges including those related to Indigenous sovereignty and human displacement (e.g., in Venezuela and Nicaragua). Occupational therapy is increasingly working in these contexts, and considering cultural explanations or developing cultural competencies is insufficient. The range of vulnerabilities these social groups experience intersects with classism, sexism, racism, political violence, and discrimination (Comisión Económica para América Latina y el Caribe, 2016). Thus, the complexity calls for an alternative way to consider neoliberalism's effects on the production of inequalities.

For instance, intercultural occupational therapy can recognize that the non-dialogues between cultural groups stem from structural, colonial, and racial divisions (Walsh, 2012). Thus, for occupational therapy, interculturality can be a tool, a process, and a professional project built organically by and with the people involved. Incorporating interculturality into professional education and occupational therapy practices can contribute as a counter-hegemonic approach to neoliberalism common sense presented by Latin American countries. For instance, those neglected Indigenous peoples' intersecting disadvantages are similar to the needs of displaced groups (e.g., Valderrama et al., 2021).

What Is Interculturality?[3]

Interculturality is a political, social, epistemic, and ethical project that aims at transforming the current relationship between cultures, which is assumed to be racialized, colonial, and instrumental to capitalism. The purpose of interculturality is the dialogue between beings, knowledge, practices, and philosophies of life to build a different society that can truly live together in harmony, valuing cultural diversity and dialogue without hegemonies (Walsh, 2012).

The emancipatory potential of intercultural health informed by Indigenous, traditional, popular knowledge and practices in a shared territory is a project in which occupational therapy can exist as a counter-hegemonic profession. Latin American history of colonization, and more recently imperialism, requires us to elaborate decolonial and anticolonial proposals to promote

3 For more information on interculturality, see Chapters 2 and 7 of this book.

structural changes related to the colonial atrocities and growing inequalities related to neoliberal ideologies (Mignolo & Walsh, 2018; Smallwood et al., 2021). For instance, how can occupational therapy contribute to the recognition and self-determination of Indigenous peoples without romanticizing or folklorizing? To respond to the question, occupational therapists must recognize that some occupations are currently at risk of extinction due to the influence of neoliberal ideologies on people's ways of living. For instance, occupations—forms of doing and shared knowledge—of Indigenous peoples are being erased (Narváez, 2021). Support for the cultural heritage of the Latin American region, including Indigenous cosmovision, should be core to the professional project to inform an alternative way to the ubiquitous neoliberalism present in the profession. This does not aim to invalidate Western scientific knowledge but to dispute its hegemony as the only possible way of constructing valuable knowledge to inform ways of living and policies (Mignolo & Walsh, 2018).

It is essential to stop the direct adoption of policies, practices, or models from countries of the Global North. The Western neoliberal practices in Latin America as a form of validation represent a "zombification" of development that impacts social, cultural, and economic structures (Brito-Alvarado & Capito, 2020). The consequence of these practices is neglecting opportunities of ways of living situated practices that can contribute to a decolonial occupational therapy. The historical belief and uncritical discourse that occupational therapy is a holistic profession do not imply that it is so in its application. As presented in previous sections of this chapter, practices within the neoliberal health sector have a role in the (re)production of oppressive power relations, colonization, neoliberalism, and cultural hegemony.

Reflections about what is next

Considering the social challenges emerging worldwide, it is evident that health professions, such as occupational therapy, cannot be neutral. Professions are built through an ethical-political positioning that defines and situates them (Lapierre, 2022a). Some occupational therapists have wanted to go further and have turned their professional practice into militancy, joining activism and advocacy movements, which have increased significantly in Chile since the outbreak of social protests in 2019 (Grandón Valenzuela, 2020; Lapierre, 2022a, 2022b). We can also see examples of this in Chile through the development of feminist collectives of female occupational therapists who seek to develop practices toward more just reproductive and women's health;[4] or colleagues who are part of groups of sexual or gender dissidence and who have promoted initiatives in the field of occupational therapy[5] that question hegemonical practices in the area of health; or Indigenous occupational therapists who work with/in Indigenous communities who have decided to form part of the Indigenous movement assuming a position at the service of an autonomous health project for Indigenous peoples and making the health professional an ally (see Quispe, 2021). The numerous social movements related to health, disability, or inclusive education have pushed professionals to take a stand and join activist groups, putting their knowledge and experience at the disposal of larger citizenship projects. Health is no longer the domain of the profession but a popular and public space for dialogue.

After the Chilean social outbreak that began on October 18, 2019,[6] resulting in a democratic, participatory, and popular constitutional reform process, many occupational therapists belonging to the private and public health systems have participated in debates and discussions in the community to decide together how to raise a justice-based healthcare system (Lapierre, 2022b). For many occupational therapists, it was the first time they experienced a secondary role in this dialogue about health, where the citizenry was the protagonist. Health professionals, including occupational therapists, are usually protagonists in debates on health and the health system, as they are valued for their professional training; however, the questions and demands on the health system that come from large social movements made up of the working class, intersectional groups, and historically excluded popular groups transform the focus of the discussion, emphasizing inequities, low participation, and everyday life (Muñoz, 2021).

In the current health and social context, it is essential to question the dominant models in health, not only to contest the system in terms of financing but also to advocate for a system that is also capable of valuing other systems of beliefs and knowledge or that can put social participation as a central axis of its health policy. As professionals, we (as a collective) are challenged to recognize the place of our profession in these struggles and contribute with proposals for health systems and policies that represent an alternative to neoliberalism, such as intercultural health centers, community

4 Such as Núcleo Feminista de Terapeutas Ocupacionales: https://nfto.cl

5 Such as Miausobreruedas: https://miausobreruedas.reservio.com

6 After the rise in public transport fares, on October 18, 2019, a popular social outbreak began in Chile with the support of almost 80% of the country, which protested against the inequity of the country. These street demonstrations lasted several months, until the start of the COVID-19 pandemic, and achieved some social changes, including the beginning of a popular process for a new Constitution.

health centers, feminist health collectives, or a system of shared responsibility care. Professionals can help to establish a permanent dialogue between the state and citizens in the health and welfare systems.

Furthermore, we must influence the state's role by closely engaging with communities and political actors. Building a profession connected to the changing reality of a society increasingly affected by neoliberal common sense requires us to be constantly aware of who we are as professional, scientific, and political actors. Occupational therapy may be a tool that contributes to reducing inequality; however, it may also be an instrument that deepens the social inequalities in a health free market. Exercising an activist and committed occupational therapy seems the only way to defend citizenship rights.

Conclusions

- Making visible and addressing the mechanisms through which neoliberalism exerts power on the profession can facilitate enacting practices that resist promoting relationships between consumers and vendors of services.
- Understanding how neoliberalism shapes professional practices and the values underpinning its way of thinking is essential to developing practices that reclaim traditional occupations.
- Anti-neoliberal professional practices are brought into light as examples that overcome the neoliberal common sense created by social inequality and a fractured public-private health system.

References

Almonacid, P., Figueroa, D., Söllner, G., & Solsona Cisternas, D. A. (2021). Terapia ocupacional ¿para todos? Su Exclusión parcial de FONASA en usuarios Pediátricos con parálisis cerebral en La Región de Magallanes, Chile. *Revista Chilena De Terapia Ocupacional, 21*(1), 67–80. https://doi.org/10.5354/0719-5346.2021.51411

Ayo, N. (2012). Understanding health promotion in a neoliberal climate and the making of health-conscious citizens. *Critical Public Health, 22*(1), 99–105. https://doi.org/10.1080/09581596.2010.520692

Bastías, G., Pantoja, T., Leisewitz, T., & Zárate, V. (2008). Health care reform in Chile. *CMAJ, 179*(12), 1289–1292.

Bezerra, W. C., & Trindade, R. L. P. (2013). A terapia ocupacional na sociedade capitalista e sua inserção profissional nas políticas sociais no Brasil. *Cadernos Brasileiros De Terapia Ocupacional, 21*(2). https://doi.org/10.4322/cto.2013.045

Bezerra, W. C., Lopes, R. E., & Basso, A. C. S. (2022). The structures of everyday life and occupational therapy: Tensioning limits and possibilities in/of the professional practice. *Cadernos Brasileiros de Terapia Ocupacional, 30*, e3031. https://doi.org/10.1590/2526-8910.ctoEN22983031

Blanchet Garneau, A., Browne, A. J., & Varcoe, C. (2019). Understanding competing discourses as a basis for promoting equity in primary health care. *BMC Health Service Research, 19*, 764. https://doi.org/10.1186/s12913-019-4602-3

Brito-Alvarado, X., & Capito, J. (2020). Neoliberalismo como necropolítica zombi. *Argumentos: Revista de Crítica Social, 22*, 252–279. https://dialnet.unirioja.es/servlet/articulo?codigo=8051262

Bushby, K., Chan, J., Druif, S., Ho, K., & Kinsella, E. A. (2015). Ethical tensions in occupational therapy practice: A scoping review. *British Journal of Occupational Therapy, 78*(4), 212–221. https://doi.org/10.1177/0308022614564770

Chomsky, N., & Waterstone, M. (2020). *Consequences of Capitalism: Manufacturing Discontent and Resistance*. Haymarket Books.

Comisión Económica para América Latina y el Caribe. (2016). *La Matriz de la Desigualdad en América Latina*. http://repositorio.cepal.org/bitstream/handle/11362/40668/S1600946_es.pdf?sequence=4&isAllowed=y

Connell, R., Fawcett, B., & Meagher, G. (2009). Neoliberalism, new public management and the human service professions: Introduction to the Special issue. *Journal of Sociology, 45*(4), 331–338. https://doi.org/10.1177/1440783309346472

da Silva, R., & Ferreira, M. (2020). Enhancing citizenship through nursing care in Brazil: Patients' struggle against austerity policies. *Nursing Inquiry, 27*(2), e12337. https://doi.org/10.1111/nin.12337

Dos Santos, V. (2022). Social transformation on the neoliberal university: Reconstructing an academic commitment. *Journal of Occupational Science, 29*(4), 482–486. https://doi.org/10.1080/14427591.2022.2110660

Durocher, E., Kinsella, E. A., McCorquodale, L., & Phelan, S. (2016). Ethical tensions related to systemic constraints: Occupational alienation in occupational therapy practice. *Occupational Therapy Journal of Research, 36*(4), 216–226. https://doi.org/10.1177/1539449216665117

Esposito, L., & Perez, F. M. (2014). Neoliberalism and the commodification of mental health. *Humanity & Society, 38*(4), 414–442. https://doi.org/10.1177/0160597614544958

Farias, K. K. R., & Bezerra, W. C. (2016). Institutional conditions and coping strategies of precarious work conditions for occupational therapists in public hospitals. *Cadernos Brasileiros De Terapia Ocupacional, 24*(2), 235–246. https://doi.org/10.4322/0104-4931.ctoAO0576

Farias, L. (2020). The (Mis)shaping of health: Problematizing neoliberal discourses of individualism and responsibility. In H. Hosseini, J. Goodman, S. C. Motta, & B. K. Gills (Eds.), *The Routledge Handbook of Transformative Global Studies* (pp. 268–281). Routledge.

Farias, L., & Aldrich, R. (2021). Critical theory: Resources for questioning and transforming everyday life. In S. Taff (Ed.), *Philosophy and Occupational Therapy: Informing Education, Research, and Practice* (pp. 155–162). Slack.

Farias, L., & Rudman, D. L. (2019). Practice analysis: Critical reflexivity on discourses constraining socially transformative occupational therapy practices. *British Journal of Occupational Therapy, 82*(11), 693–697. https://doi.org/10.1177/0308022619862111

Fischer, K. (2009). The influence of neoliberals in Chile before, during, and after Pinochet. In P. Mirowski & D. Plehwe (Eds.), *The Road from Mont Pèlerin: The Making of the Neoliberal Thought Collective* (pp. 305–346). Harvard University Press.

Foucault, M. (1977). Technologies of the self. In P. Rabinow (Ed.), *Michel Foucault: Ethics, Subjectivity and Truth: The Essential Works of Foucault, Vol. 1*. The New Press.

Göttems, L. B. D., & Mollo, M. L. R. (2020). Neoliberalism in Latin America: Effects on health system reforms. *Revista de Saúde Pública, 54*, 74. https://doi.org/10.11606/s1518-8787.2020054001806

Grandón Valenzuela, D. (2019). Función económica de las ocupaciones feminizadas no remuneradas: Una crítica desde la economía feminista. *Revista Ocupación Humana, 18*(2), 54–67. https://doi.org/10.25214/25907816.228

Grandón Valenzuela, D. (2020). Negar la cotidianidad: Una propuesta epistémica para la Terapia Ocupacional a partir de una autoetnografía de la revuelta popular en Chile. *Revista Ocupación Humana, 20*(2), 25–46. https://latinjournal.org/index.php/roh/article/view/881/805

Hammell, K. R. W. (2016). Empowerment and occupation: A new perspective. *Canadian Journal of Occupational Therapy, 83*(5), 281–287. https://doi.org/10.1177/0008417416652910

Harvey, D. (2007). *A Brief History of Neoliberalism*. Oxford University Press.

Hayes, K., Dos Santos, V., Costigan, M., & Morante, D. (2023). Extension, austerity, and emergence: Themes identified from a global scoping review of non-urban occupational therapy services. *Australian Occupational Therapy Journal, 70*(1), 142–156. https://doi.org/10.1111/1440-1630.12844

Herrera Sandoval, M., & Valderrama Nuñez, C. (2013). Gubernamentalidad y biopolítica: Una aproximación con los saberes y prácticas históricas de la terapia ocupacional en Chile. *Revista Chilena de Terapia Ocupacional, 13*(2), 79–92. https://doi.org/10.5354/0719-5346.2013.30218

Hokowhitu, B. (2014). If you are not healthy, then what are you? Healthism, colonial disease and body-logic. In K. Fitzpatrick & R. Tinning (Eds.), *Health Education: Critical Perspectives*. Routledge.

Húmeres, M. (2017). Hacia una genealogía del niño símbolo. In O. Pavez (Ed.), *Des(orden) de Género: Políticas y Mercados del Cuerpo en Chile* (pp. 279–298). Crann Editores.

Irvine-Brown, L., Ware, V.-A., & Malfitano, A. P. S. (2022). Exploring the praxis of occupational therapy-community development practitioners. *Canadian Journal of Occupational Therapy, 89*(1), 26–35. https://doi.org/10.1177/00084174211066662

Kincheloe, J. L., & McLaren, P. (2005). Rethinking critical theory and qualitative research. In N. K. Denzin & Y. S. Lincoln (Eds.), *Handbook of Qualitative Research, Vol. 3* (pp. 303–342). Sage.

Lapierre, M. (2020). Análisis del sistema de salud chileno desde una perspectiva de justicia, en el marco del movimiento social del 18 de Octubre de 2019 en Chile. *Revista Izquierdas,* (49), 4384–4403. www.izquierdas.cl/images/pdf/2020/n49/art207_4384_4403.pdf

Lapierre, M. (2022a). Decolonialidad e interculturalidad como lugares de enunciación para analizar la terapia ocupacional en Chile. In V. Dos Santos, I. Muñoz, & M. Farias (Eds.), *Cuestiones y Prácticas Contemporáneas de la Terapia Ocupacional en América del Sur* (pp. 53–60). Editora CRV.

Lapierre, M. (2022b). La terapia ocupacional en el agitado escenario sociopolítico del Chile actual [Letter to the editor]. *Revista ContexTO, 8*, 13–16. https://revistacontextoucen.cl/index.php/contexto/article/download/34/25

Lecours, A., Baril, N., & Drolet, M.-J. (2021). What is professionalism in occupational therapy? A concept analysis. *Canadian Journal of Occupational Therapy, 88*(2), 117–130. https://doi.org/10.1177/0008417421994377

Lopes, R. E., & de Oliveira Borba, P. L. (2022). A inclusão radical como diretriz para terapeutas ocupacionais na educação. *Revista Ocupación Humana, 22*(2), 202–227.

Loveman, B. (1986). Military dictatorship and political opposition in Chile, 1973–1986. *Journal of Interamerican Studies and World Affairs, 28*(4), 1–38. https://doi.org/10.2307/165745

Mignolo, W. D., & Walsh, C. (2018). *On Decoloniality: Concepts, Analytics, Praxis*. Duke University Press.

Ministerio de Desarrollo Social [Ministry of Social Development]. (2018). *CASEN 2017: Salud-Síntesis de Resultados*. Santiago de Chile: Observatorio Social-Ministerio de Desarrollo Social. https://observatorio.ministeriodesarrollosocial.gob.cl/storage/docs/casen/2017/Resultados_Salud_casen_2017.pdf

Missoni, E., & Solimano, G. (2010). *Towards Universal Health Coverage: The Chilean Experience*. World Health Report, Background Paper 4. https://cdn.who.int/media/docs/default-source/health-financing/technical-briefs-background-papers/4chile.pdf

Molina, C., & Tobar, F. (2018). ¿Qué significa Neoliberalismo en salud? *Revista De Ciencias Sociales y Humanas, 12*(12), 65–73. www.ojs.unsj.edu.ar/index.php/reviise/article/view/272

Muñoz, C. G. (2021). Pandemia y estallido social en Chile: La acción social vinculada a las demandas de salud. In C. Tetelboin, D. Iturrieta, & C. Schor-Landman (Eds.), *América Latina: Sociedad, Política y Salud en Tiempos de Pandemias* (pp. 177–191). CLASCO.

Narváez, S. E. (2021). Terapia ocupacional y cultura: Reflexiones sobre una experiencia con artesanos tradicionales de las provincias de San Juan y Salta. *Revista Argentina de Terapia Ocupacional, 7*(2), 80–87. https://revista.terapia-ocupacional.org.ar/index.php/rato_2022/article/view/162

Navarro, V. (2008). Neoliberalism and its consequences: The world health situation since Alma Ata. *Global Social Policy, 8*(2), 152–155.

Ong, A. (2007). Neoliberalism as a mobile technology. *Transactions of the Institute of British Geographers, 32*(1), 3–8. www.jstor.org/stable/4639996

Owens, J., Singh, G., & Cribb, A. (2019). Austerity and professionalism: Being a good healthcare professional in bad conditions. *Health Care Analysis, 27*, 157–170. https://doi.org/10.1007/s10728-019-00372-y

Peacock, M., Bissell, P., & Owen, J. (2014). Dependency denied: Health inequalities in the neo-liberal era. *Social Science & Medicine, 118*, 173–180. https://doi.org/10.1016/j.socscimed.2014.08.006

Pérez, L. O. (2021). *Ocupación Humana: De la Matriz Colonial Moderna Hacia la Construcción de Saberes Sociales del Sur*. Facultad de Medicina. Universidad Nacional de Colombia.

Pizarro, E., Estrella, S., Figueroa, F., Helmke, F., Pontigo, C., & Whiteford, G. (2018). Understanding occupational justice from the concept of territory: A proposal for occupational science. *Journal of Occupational Science, 25*(4), 463–473. https://doi.org/10.1080/14427591.2018.1487261

Prado, A. C. da S. A., Silva, C. R., & Silvestrini, M. S. (2020). Juventudes, trabalho e cultura em tempos de racionalidade neoliberal. *Cadernos Brasileiros De Terapia Ocupacional, 28*(2), 706–724. https://doi.org/10.4322/2526-8910.ctoARF1846

Quispe, J. (2021). *Cosmovisiõn Aymara: Un Acercamiento para Profesionales de la Salud*. Universidad Antofagasta; EDISEA. https://fliphtml5.com/zalyb/qnmn/basic

Reina Bolaños, C. A. (2021). El sistema de salud colombiano: Reflexiones sobre su influencia en la salud de la población. *Revista Ocupación Humana, 21*(2), 88–98. https://doi.org/10.25214/25907816.911

Rodríguez, J. P. (2021). The politics of neoliberalism in Latin America: Dynamics of resilience and contestation. *Sociology Compass, 15*(3), e12854. https://doi.org/10.1111/soc4.12854

Rolack Jaramillo, S., Triviños Rubilar, V., & Troncoso Henriquez, P. (2015). La influencia del sistema neoliberal en las elecciones ocupacionales y el impacto en la salud y bienestar desde una perspectiva cualitativa. *Revista Chilena de Terapia Ocupacional, 15*(2). https://doi.org/10.5354/0719-5346.2015.38168

Rose, N. (2013). Personalized medicine: Promises, problems and perils of a new paradigm for healthcare. *Procedia – Social and Behavioral Sciences, 77*, 341–352. https://doi.org/10.1016/j.sbspro.2013.03.092

Rotarou, E. S., & Sakellariou, D. (2017). Neoliberal reforms in health systems and the construction of long-lasting inequalities in health care: A case study from Chile. *Health Policy, 121*(5), 495–503. https://doi.org/10.1016/j.healthpol.2017.03.005

Rottenberg, C. (2018). Neoliberal meritocracy. *Cultural Studies, 32*(6), 997–999. https://doi.org/10.1080/09502386.2018.1435703

Rudman, D. L. (2013). Enacting the critical potential of occupational science: Problematizing the "individualizing of occupation." *Journal of Occupational Science, 20*(4), 298–313. https://doi.org/10.1080/14427591.2013.803434

Sakellariou, D., & Pollard, N. (2017). *Occupational Therapies Without Borders: Integrating Justice with Practice*. Elsevier Science.

Sakellariou, D., & Rotarou, E. S. (2017). The effects of neoliberal policies on access to healthcare for people with disabilities. *International Journal for Equity in Health, 16*(1), 199. https://doi.org/10.1186/s12939-017-0699-3

Silvestrini, M. S., Silva, C. R., & Almeida Prado, A. C. da S. (2019). Terapia ocupacional e cultura: Dimensões ético-políticas e resistências. *Cadernos Brasileiros De Terapia Ocupacional, 27*(4), 929–940. https://doi.org/10.4322/2526-8910.ctoARF1727

Smallwood, R., Woods, C., Power, T., & Usher, K. (2021). Understanding the impact of historical trauma due to colonization on the health and well-being of Indigenous young peoples: A systematic scoping review. *Journal of Transcultural Nursing, 32*(1), 59–68. https://doi.org/10.1177/1043659620935955

Stillerman, J. (2012). Chile's forgotten consumers: Poor urban families, consumption strategies, and the moral economy of risk in Santiago. In J. Sinclair & A. C. Pertierra (Eds.), *Consumer Culture in Latin America* (pp. 67–79). Palgrave Macmillan. https://doi.org/10.1057/9781137116864_5

Turcotte, P.-L., & Holmes, D. (2021). From domestication to imperial patronage: Deconstructing the biomedicalisation of occupational therapy. *Health, 27*(5), 719–737. https://doi.org/10.1177/13634593211067891

Unger, J. P., De Paepe, P., Cantuarias, G. S., & Herrera, O. A. (2008). Chile's neoliberal health reform: An assessment and a critique. *PLoS Medicine, 5*(4), e79. https://doi.org/10.1371/journal.pmed.0050079

Valderrama Núñez, C. M., Sepúlveda Hernández, S., & Hermosilla Alarcón, A. (2021). Collective occupations and nature: Impacts of the coloniality of nature on rural and fishing communities in Chile. *Journal of Occupational Science, 29*(2), 252–262. https://doi.org/10.1080/14427591.2021.1880264

Venegas Villascan, M. A., & Feregrino Feregrino, J. (2022). Fragmentación de la gobernanza en salud: Desigualdad y precarización laboral en los profesionales de la salud. *Administración y Organizaciones, 25*(48), 89–105. https://doi.org/10.24275/uam/xoc/dcsh/rayo/2022v25n48/Feregrino

Walsh, C. (2012). Interculturalidad y (de)colonialidad: Perspectivas críticas y políticas. *Visao Global, 15*(1–2), 61–74. https://dialnet.unirioja.es/servlet/articulo?codigo=5478661

CHAPTER 9

Revelations

INTERCULTURAL TRANSLATIONS IN OCCUPATIONAL THERAPY

Daniela Castro de Jong, Margarita Mondaca, Lisette Farias, and Ana Marques

Abstract

Within its century of existence, occupational therapy has been building a body of knowledge that has privileged a Global North-based perspective, portraying the *social* in occupational therapy as an exotic notion that seems to be confined to or belonging to Global South practices situated at the margins of the anglophone world. These Global North assumptions have been assumed as universal and "normalized" worldwide, resulting in recent questioning of the cultural relevance of this dominant scholarship and worldview. In this chapter, four Latin American occupational therapists reflect on what we have seen as some of the possibilities for occupational therapy based on our learning, living, and working experiences in the Global South and North. We first present how the social is understood as part of occupational therapy and knowledge construction and situate our experiences in Latin America's socioeconomic and historical contexts. Then, we illustrate how this understanding of the social often conflicts with Northern standards of knowledge and theoretical models that tend to limit the social to a dimension of individuals and consequently exoticize social, community, and collaborative approaches within occupational therapy practices. To illustrate these potential tensions, we use the concept of intercultural translations to favor alliances among Global North and South perspectives. Finally, throughout the chapter, we present guiding questions, vignettes, and personal reflections so readers can continue this dialogue in their own contexts.

Keywords
colonialism; Global North; Global South; intercultural translations; neoliberalism

Learning outcomes

- Discuss the limitations a hegemonic idea of the social has had for the occupational therapy profession.
- Explore what Global Southern perspectives add to occupational therapy practices and education in Anglophone/Global Northern contexts to address social issues of relevance to occupational therapy.
- Identify some possibilities for intercultural translation as a tool for collaboration in occupational therapy.

Introduction

Theoretical and professional growth allows us to discuss how the *social* in occupational therapy has been delimited and associated with *Southern* perspectives. Just by looking at a common definition of the word "social" by the Spanish Royal Academy, it is seen as something that is part of or belongs to a society/company, about a given jurisdictional order, or related to the less favored economic classes (Real Academia Española, n.d.). This gives a first indication of why and how the social might be connected as something that matters in the South. The need for looking deeper at the idea of the social in occupational therapy is an overlooked and taken-for-granted dimension within knowledge creation and practices in the profession. Understanding what the social is and represents goes beyond the profession of occupational therapy. The social can be characterized by how we live together in society intersected by diverse dynamics of privilege/marginalization determining and infused in everyday practices (Granda, 2004). In this sense, the attention to the social developed by critical occupational therapy practices in the South (e.g., Galheigo, 2011; Guajardo & Mondaca, 2017) is a political response of the profession to varied forms of suffering and a striving toward social justice and social transformation by acknowledging and reducing the oppressing conditions.

For instance, in Brazil, the social has been defined in relation to a critique of the conception of therapeutic activity as discussed by Galheigo et al. (2018, p. 731) looking at the ideas of Nascimento (1990), who proposed moving toward the idea of "viewing it as a therapeutic instrument and mechanistic resource of healing according to a scientific standpoint to understanding activity as an element of culture, polysemous and complex, based on a sociopolitical and affective dimension of the human condition." From this perspective, a materialist-historical framework of occupational therapy (Francisco, 1988) emerged, which has broadened the concept of activity to integrate different types of doing such as opportunities for coexistence and sociability, collective organization, and social participation, among others (Galheigo et al., 2018). Guajardo (2016) expands on this idea by emphasizing the need for a Southern history within occupational therapy. This history should place local practices in connection with the socioeconomic and cultural issues impacting the doing of local communities by acknowledging the profession's commitment to respect for freedom (Guajardo, 2016). Understanding occupation in an ahistorical and not situated manner would then deny the social and ignore critical issues for practice.

Valderrama (2019) claims that occupational therapy practices in the Global South can only occur in the social arena. This is where individuals and communities live, express their emotions, mourn, and navigate despair. As a result of this, occupational therapy in Latin America, as in other areas of the world (Jansen van Vuuren, Okyere, & Aldersey, 2020), is ruled by neoliberal socioeconomies, and, therefore, cannot ignore how it has developed immersed in social and health inequalities (Meyers & Hunt, 2014). Very recently, Ana Malfitano, in her keynote presentation at the 2022 World Federation of Occupational Therapists Conference, called our attention to the social nature of our work (Malfitano, 2022). However, the social nature of occupational therapy has not been fully articulated. From a historical materialist perspective (Vidal, 1988), social life, in all its nuances in everyday life, is a product of the material conditions and the forms of relationships created by a given society's socioeconomic and political frameworks.

Incorporating a social and human-rights perspective has been characteristic in occupational therapy practices in the South, and therefore not delimited to theoretical aspects promoted from the North (Guajardo, Kronenberg, & Ramugondo, 2015). Within this ethical and human-rights perspective, social justice is understood as the equal distribution of social rights (Guajardo, 2020). Thus, the articulation of the social is becoming an urgent matter to respond to the needs of those facing social challenges in everyday life, such as situations of armed conflict, the decline of welfare across Europe, and forced migration across the globe, to name a few. These challenges require a debate about the role and responsibility of the profession in social issues that affect people's conditions to participate in society. Even though current and emerging social challenges have brought to life issues for consideration in the professional actions in the Global North, this is in direct tension with the call from evidence-based and individualistic approaches in practice (Taff & Putnam, 2022).

As professionals, we are asked to carefully examine our roles and how practices and educational strategies support occupational therapists' responses to global challenges. To facilitate this discussion, we propose using *intercultural translations*[1] (de Sousa Santos, 2014) to learn about the underlying assumptions among Global South and North perspectives and develop intercommunication that strengthens the work of occupational therapists for social justice and human dignity. As a first step, we will position ourselves, then we will go on to define what we mean by Global North and Global South and contextualize our point of departure: Latin America. Then, we will explore key concepts such as colonization and neoliberalism. This will be followed by our discussions and reflections around the experiences of doing and working as occupational therapists in the Global North. By the end of the chapter, we propose an applied exploration of the concept of intercultural translations (de Sousa Santos, 2014).

Positionality

This chapter was written by four occupational therapists who recognize themselves as locals in several territories, including Europe, Latin America, and Australia. This chapter presents the reflections of these four co-authors whose first language is not English and whose personal and professional experiences have been shaped by growing up and/or practicing under military dictatorships or their aftermath. It is worth noting that our discussions do not represent the experiences of all Latin American occupational therapists working and living in the Global North or South.

DC: With multiple migration experiences within my family, I always thought it would be my time to do so one day. I left Chile after 20 years of practice in academic, pediatric, gerontology, and community settings. My first stop was Sweden to pursue my doctoral studies, and then Australia, where I work as an academic and researcher. Has it been easy? Definitely not. Has it been worth it? Absolutely yes. After over a decade of wandering around the world and wondering who I am as an occupational therapist, I finally understood that I might no longer be physically in the Global South. However, it is with me in everything I do. From my tolerance to uncertainty to solidarity, and by holding my deep belief in the idea that we are because we belong.

1 De Sousa Santos (2014) defines intercultural translations as "searching for isomorphic concerns and underlying assumptions among cultures, identifying differences and similarities, and developing, whenever appropriate, new hybrid forms of cultural understanding and intercommunication that may be useful in favouring interactions and strengthening alliances among social movements fighting...against capitalism, colonialism, and patriarchy and for social justice, human dignity, and human decency" (p. 212).

MM: I was trained and worked clinically and in academia for 20 years in Chile in human rights and mental health. The period during and after dictatorship in Latin American countries forged the practices of occupational therapy and the profession's territories within the social. The Chilean dictatorship left physical and mental health wounds among our population and installed a strong and rigid neoliberal socioeconomic system, creating dramatic health and social inequalities. These inequalities were part of the conditions where occupational therapy in Chile articulated and developed its practices. This understanding of occupational therapy grounded in human rights has been my compass when moving and practicing in European academia.

LF: I studied occupational therapy in Chile, in a public university, to later study for a master's in Europe and a Ph.D. in Canada. This international background has made me reflect on the different economic systems and social expectations that shape our work and how we respond to specific trends through education and practice. Before studying occupational therapy, I volunteered in deprived areas on the outskirts of Santiago, particularly with children affected by socio-disadvantaged conditions. Then I worked in children's rehabilitation in a public hospital in Chile. These experiences in the public sector left several footprints in my work today, which mainly focuses on critical health research and transformative practice.

AM: Before and throughout my occupational therapy training, I volunteered in a shelter for children. Once I graduated, I developed these experiences by working in a social day center and being part of the Metuia Project.[2] Then I came to France as an undocumented migrant, working and being hosted by family or friends. However, I did not think about it until it was necessary to address these experiences methodologically to understand their impact on the occupational therapist I am today.

Global North and Global South

It is worth noticing that the terms *Global North* and *Global South* are used in this chapter based on de Sousa Santos' (2014) conceptualization that goes beyond geographical location and the imaginary line dividing European powers from their colonies. Previously called the third or fourth

2 Research laboratory in Brazil where we have developed community projects, teaching occupational therapy for the undergraduate students; researching in undergraduate (honors thesis), master's, and Ph.D. levels, about subjects related to social occupational therapy actions with people experiencing disadvantageous social conditions.

world, the so-called Global South was presented as geographically disconnected from the Northern societies by the "Brandt Line," which divided the world into North and South, becoming a recognizable and influential representation of the economic and political division of both worlds (Lees, 2021).

De Sousa Santos (2014) states that the Global North and South are coexisting and maintain given beliefs and worldviews that are embedded within power-relation dynamics. This is further explained by Meyers and Hunt (2014) and their consideration of local South areas, regions, or even neighborhoods in Global North countries. This ongoing relationship—in local and global terms—continues to oppress and marginalize groups (denominated as South) by imposing the consequences of capitalism and privileging elites that benefit from it (the North) (de Sousa Santos, 2014). An example of this can be found in the work of Gonçalves and Malfitano (2020) as they presented the lived experience of young Brazilians living in a favela (a local South within a country in which the richest 5% have the same income as the remaining 95%). Beyond the experiences of living in poverty, sense of identity, and extended stigmatization of those living in the favela, the participants reported the impact on common occupations, such as urban mobility (Gonçalves & Malfitano, 2020). Regardless of where we are situated, it is important to consider the Glocal (Global + Local) continuum (Correia et al., 2021).

Consistent with de Sousa Santos' (2014) as well as Meyers and Hunt's (2014) ideas, our reflections are not based on geographical divisions but are an attempt to illustrate how the global spread of capitalism, characterized by an increase in social inequities and conditions of vulnerability for particular groups (Harvey, 2005; Zhang, Andrew, & Rudkin, 2012) in Northern and Southern societies, has introduced the need for looking deeper at the social in occupational therapy from different perspectives.

Vignette 1: When the Global South is Invisible on the Occupational Therapy Map

Different authors from the Global South, such as Correia et al. (2021), Guajardo (2020), and Valderrama (2019), explored the idea of colonization in our professional knowledge. Through this process, Southern ways of knowing remain invisible for the larger professional community. Duarte Cuervo and Talero Cabrejo (2022) expand on this, including the impact on knowledge production and translation.

This phenomenon is prevalent and can be seen through the following:

- Assuming universality of a specific set of values and knowledge from the Global North.
- Denial of local realities and languages in education.
- Forcing complex phenomena into standardized and evidence-based approaches.
- The pursuit of "scientific" truth. If we are not scientific in a Global North way, we will not belong and will remain invisible on the map.

Latin America as the point of departure

While the region shares a vast territory below the Rio Bravo (across the border between Mexico and the USA), it cannot be seen as a monolithic entity either or across countries (Bianchi & Malfitano, 2022; Dos Santos, 2017). The diversity comes from how each country in the region has dealt with other commonalities, such as natural disasters, political instability, corruption, and structural violence (Bianchi & Malfitano, 2022; Dos Santos, 2017).

According to the Organisation for Economic Co-operation and Development (OECD, 2020), before the COVID-19 pandemic one in five people lived in absolute poverty in Latin America (i.e., income insufficient to meet basic needs such as food or shelter). There was a sharp increase in poverty and a slight increase in income inequality in 2020, which declined in 2021, but not by enough to fully reverse the negative effects of the pandemic (e.g., Latin America's poverty rate reached 32.3% in 2021) (CEPAL, 2022). Poverty is not a new phenomenon in the region. Since colonialization, an elite of upper-class European descent has monopolized resources and privileges, including access to private healthcare and education, and ownership of land or *haciendas*,[3] the system of landowners, and Indigenous labor (Beghin, 2022). This legacy of colonialism was reinforced by the implementation of neoliberal socioeconomic and political systems across the region, maintaining these social inequalities for generations in the context of weak state protection, creating the condition for what Beghin (2022) described as "an unequal, racist, and sexist region that destroys natural resources" (p. 179).

The social nature of life in Latin America

Everyday occupations in Latin America can then be understood (or misunderstood) through widely spread images or stereotypes. The region is

3 Large pieces of land often controlled by one family with several servants working in plantations.

usually identified by its festive, laid-back, and friendly attitude. However, these images are also associated with corruption, drug-dealing, violence, and poverty through commercial films and shows. The region remains an exotic land where *everything* (even anything) is possible.

Considering that the socioeconomic and political framework of the 21st century is grounded in extracting resources and destruction of lands-beings-knowledges, with an emphasis in the subjugation of Latin American and Indigenous perspectives (Mignolo & Walsh, 2018), occupational therapy is called to articulate responsive practices grounded in the respect and promotion of human rights (Guajardo & Mondaca, 2017) and acknowledgement of the inner holism of traditional forms of knowledge.

Vignette 2: We Call the Mexican Wave... the Wave; we call Social Occupational Therapy... Occupational Therapy

In the Global South (and anywhere else), we must—carefully and respectfully—learn from and acknowledge our lived experiences, our centennial Indigenous heritages, our unstable economies and political systems, our breathtaking landscapes and natural disasters, our shared history of brutal colonization (still alive through coloniality). Acknowledging this will allow us to further understand the conditions and probably the needs from which occupational therapy needs to respond through the local practices in the region. These needs and conditions will appear in terms of social issues. These issues are not emerging on a given day; social issues are expressed in our daily life, every single day. Forcing foreign given ways of living, conceptual models of practice, and evidence from the Global North becomes somehow retraumatizing. Moreover, the Global North is now facing the emergence of similar phenomena with no response from the more individualistic approaches. Our work as a discipline in that space in the Global North has been labeled as "social" occupational therapy (which differs from the conceptualization proposed by Brazilian occupational therapists) as if our actions were not embedded in and defined socially. In Latin America in our daily practices, dealing with vulnerability, poverty, or exclusion is what we call occupational therapy, no labels needed.

Diverse forms of colonization

In Latin America, the colonization processes, and the influence of coloniality[4] (Beghin, 2022; Maldonado-Torres, 2007), globalization, and neoliberalism, continue to shape the extreme inequalities experienced by large social groups. Globalization, colonialism, and capitalism gained new forms, such as neoliberalism. While Latin America is mainly in the geographical South, it is also part of the political, cultural, and economic Global South. The Global South is about the unbalanced power relationships between the mainstream metropoles (Europe and North America) and the world's peripheries (Connell, 2007). As a result of the unbalanced power, the Global South remains marginalized (Connell, 2007). De Sousa Santos (2014) expands on this idea, acknowledging that this is replicated locally in Latin America, creating conditions for social inequality. These relationships are shaped by a power imbalance, exclusion, knowledge dominance, and appropriation (Connell, 2007; de Sousa Santos, 2014).

Reflection 1: Reflect on Your Understanding of Human Doing

- How is your understanding of human occupation shaped by your family history, context, and socioeconomic conditions?
- Do you see human occupation as embedded within the person who engages in it? Or embedded within a social network of conditions that shape it?
- Have you encountered occupational therapists from other countries or regions? Have you noticed some commonalities and differences in the approaches and practices?

Cognitive justice reminds us of how dominant ways of knowing imposed by colonization have dismissed what is considered knowledge outside their dominant empires (Visvanathan, 1997). The impact of this imposition on alternative non-Northern forms of knowledge meant that people's lifestyles and sets of beliefs were denominated as "primitive," exotic, not legitimate, or irrelevant to the development of their societies. This includes, but is not limited to, Indigenous ways of knowing. Yakushko (2018) explains this

4 Coloniality represents the continuity of power patterns resulting from historical colonialism characterized by foreign territorial occupation but covering bodies and minds as a mode of domination, within the scope of work, culture, intersubjective relationships, identities, and the production of knowledge (Maldonado-Torres, 2007).

through the exploration of how, because of colonization, traditional knowledges from healers and shamans were dismissed and oppressed. Another example is presented by Garzón López (2013) in terms of how Indigenous knowledges in the region were suppressed and denied as the Eurocentric views were seen as unquestionable. In this line, de Sousa Santos (2007) also employs the term cognitive justice to argue the dominant privilege of Global North science that hinders a dialogue between diverse knowledges in a professional level. For occupational therapists in the Global South, Guajardo et al. (2015) call them to work toward cognitively just recognition of the ways of knowing present in the region which existed before colonial times.

Neoliberalism

The impact and effects of globalization and colonialism cannot be understood without looking at neoliberalism. Mignolo (2021) reminds us:

> [...] what has all this to do with globalization? Everything. Globalization isn't just trade, transportation, fast cybernetic interconnections, the sale of information, and all manner of things material and aethereal you could add to the list. Or better yet, globalization IS thought to be all of that, packaged in the language of progress and civilization, buzzwords of the West until WWII, of modernization and development recalling the talk of the fifties and sixties, and our lingo since the eighties of development and market democracy, the last chapter of the long story of Westernization: the neoliberal story of globalization. (p. 727)

Neoliberalism is a sociopolitical and economic system and governing logic that organizes societies and economies around the principle of free-market activity, shifting the balance of power toward dominant economic classes that control market activity (Harvey, 2005).

Neoliberalism is a powerful force shaping economies and societies in ways that perpetuate colonialism by the dominant economic groups by promoting values such as individualism, consumerism, competition, and meritocracy (Farias, 2020; Harvey, 2005). These values and logic have presented challenges to those inherited by previous collective cultural traditions by perpetuating individualism and competition (Farias, 2020). By supporting commercial liberty and entrepreneurial freedom, neoliberalism incentivizes private investment, such as private schools or clinics, promoting the idea of free choice and free markets (Farias, 2020).

This economic system and logic were first introduced in Chile as an experiment in the context of the military dictatorship[5] during the early 1980s. This neoliberal experiment included reforms in the Chilean healthcare system, which began with the privatization of healthcare and education (Rotarou & Sakellariou, 2017). This, combined with a history of human rights violations, unstable democracies, and racism, has created an environment in which corporate interests and local ruling classes have built on the relations of subordination and discrimination initiated during colonial rule (Quijano, 2007). Thus, neoliberalism has helped to reproduce and reshape the racial, sexual, political, and epistemological hierarchies of the colonial past that established the supposed superiority of European-based empires. For instance, with the adoption of the neoliberal model, and the flexibilization and deregulation of labor, with a consequent increase in unemployment and underemployment of the working class, precariousness of employment and disengagement not only from their jobs but also from workers and political organizations have emerged (Rodríguez, 2021).

According to the Chilean sociologist Rodríguez (2021), the most prominent questions for scholars and professionals today are how alternative strategies to neoliberalism can be developed, what this could mean for the relationship between the state and the market, and which institutions and actors (professional groups, activists, and communities) should contribute to developing these alternatives. Max-Neef (2010), in his talk at the World Federation of Occupational Therapists Conference held in Chile, asked occupational therapists to critically reflect on the need for anti-neoliberal alternatives. His call was especially relevant in the context of privatization of healthcare services and education in Latin America (Max-Neef, 2010).

The introduction of neoliberal reforms in Latin America led to dramatic changes in the field of education. For example, when most of this chapter's co-authors studied occupational therapy, there were no private universities in Chile offering this program. Most occupational therapists graduated from one public university in Chile (on the only program between the early 1960s and late 1990s). However, by 2022, there were eight approved and 16 non-approved programs in occupational therapy in Chile with several hundred graduates each year (WFOT, 2022) who need to secure a job in a free market that tends to employ as many people as possible at the expense of reducing job guarantees, union protection, and other labor rights (Rotarou & Sakellariou, 2017). This neoliberal free market also demands effectiveness by pressuring professionals to compete and justify the need for one's position within private institutions (Owens, Singh, & Cribb, 2019). In this way, occupational

5 For more information about the military dictatorship that affected Chile during 1973–1986, see Loveman (1986).

therapy students might be subjects of a paradox on which they learn about the dramatic impact of neoliberalism in people's occupations while their own higher-education experience is defined and ruled by it. In this sense, occupational therapists are immersed in a neoliberal capitalist framework from the beginning of their training, dictating their professional conditions and impeding addressing the roots of social and health inequalities.

Reflection 2: When the Social Is at Your Front Door—Exploring Homelessness as a Lived Experience That Is Highly Shaped by the Social

One of the co-authors has worked with homeless people in France since 2004. Through their work they identified the impact of the surrounding contexts on people's daily life activities, limiting access to rights and social participation. They proposed that working on these activities was a way to improve their daily life, in connection with the public policies related to this population, as identified in occupational therapy literature (Galvani et al., 2016). But the local occupational therapy systems and approaches could not see its place in the action with this population. This issue has already been acknowledged in the experiences of immigrants and others in a situation of social vulnerability (Castel, 1995). When local occupational therapists propose moving the discussions on the social from practice to academia, the Global North referred them back to Brazil, as experiences of exclusion and social life are not relevant or are dramatically different in their contexts. This can be contested as precariousness has continued to rise since the end of the 1990s in France (as in other countries), particularly with the interweaving of problems of education, employment, housing, and health (Fassin, 2004; Marques, 2010; Paugam, 1996). The recent health crisis due to the pandemic impacted the most those who were in situations of vulnerability, regardless of their location. The lack of access to health and education services, as well as the lack of opportunity to exercise their rights, were evident for them. This is not new, as Bourdieu (1993) has already shown in *La Misère du Monde*[6] or Castel (1995) in *La Métamorphose de la Question Sociale.*[7] Some recent research comparing Brazil and France highlights the impact of social inequalities in citizenship in both countries (Marques & Deranty, 2017; Xypas & Wallenhorst, 2020).

6 The Misery of the World.
7 The Metamorphosis of the Social Question.

Vignette 3: We Are a Political Profession

Olivares-Aising (2018) proposes an articulation between Max-Neef's seminal work on the theory of human-scale development and occupational therapy:

- Globalization has become a tool for capitalism. When global indicators are used to assess economic status and quality of life across all contexts, without considering local characteristics and needs, they impose a singular worldview that defines what counts as progress or well-being. Other ways of understanding and measuring quality of life are rendered invisible or irrelevant.
- The Human Scale Development theory is oriented to highlight quality (over quantity) development for all. By focusing on quality, everyone can actively participate in their existence by acknowledging what matters to them (such as cultural traditions and ways of living).
- Monoculturalism in occupational therapy (the illusion of having only one culture) assigns power and privilege to a few and (in)advertently dismisses other ways of doing, experienced as inequality and marginalization.

Based on Olivares-Aising's (2018) ideas, consider the following:

- How do you think the values promoted by neoliberalism and dominant economic approaches such as capitalism may affect the sense of community or group in a determined context?
- How are economic models shaping our professional practice and communities' daily lives?
- Have you considered the idea of monoculturalism in occupational therapy before?

Learning and doing occupational therapy in the Global North while coming from the South

To explain our processes of negotiation and adjustment to the lived realities of the Global North, we propose the use of intercultural translations as defined by de Sousa Santos (2014). In the case of occupational therapy, intercultural translations cannot be understood as disconnected from the profession's rich and diverse history in Latin America. These connections are shaped by the ongoing negotiations of the local realities and practices with the notions of critical thinking versus the more technical approaches in the profession. These approaches from the Global North maintain an underlying aim for universalism and individualism, ignoring how contextual issues are responsible for social exclusion, stress, and illness (Hammell, 2021).

As Castro, Dahlin-Ivanoff, and Mårtensson (2014) described, we are at a crossroads regarding how the profession understands culture. On one road, the Northern ideas on culture prevail and nothing changes in our practice. The other road brings an invitation to critically examine how the idea of culture in occupational therapy practices developed in the Global South, which then poses a challenge of taken-for-granted assumptions (Castro et al., 2014). But this road is not only one, as the South is not a hegemonic or linear idea (Correia et al., 2021). This second road has been identified in the Global North literature as part of the emerging practices and knowledge development. For example, a Global North professional statement about diversity states that:

> [O]ther fields such as social work and education have advanced valuable alternative approaches such as anti-oppressive and emancipatory practices (Baines, 2011; Freire, 1970; Rancière, 1991). These have not yet been taken up in the occupational therapy literature. (Occupational Therapy Professional Alliance of Canada, 2014, p. 2)

Anti-oppressive and emancipatory practices have been part of occupational therapy practices in Latin America for decades (Dos Santos, 2017). Why Global South ways of doing and knowing have not been seen might be the result of a combination of complex issues, such as language barriers, embedded colonialism, changes in the living conditions in the Global North, etc. (Magalhães et al., 2019).

Below we share examples from our learning and practices in the South, in which we present some issues around intercultural translations:

An example from Brazil: Occupational therapists who actively participated in the struggles for the re-democratization of Brazil in the 1970s and 80s produced knowledge based on historical materialism and territorial community practices: social occupational therapy, occupational therapy in mental health, and occupational therapy in community-based rehabilitation. Social occupational therapy refers to politically and ethically framed practices that target individuals, groups, or systems to enable justice and social rights for people and groups experiencing disadvantageous social conditions (Barros, Ghirardi, & Lopes, 2002), which prevents them from exercising their citizenship and social participation. An example of social occupational therapy in practice is The Metuia Project. The project was created in 1998 by three professors from different universities in São Paulo, Brazil: Denise Dias Barros, Roseli Esquerdo Lopes, and Sandra Galheigo. From there it has expanded to other higher-education institutions across the country. Currently the project's goal is to continue linking practice, teaching, and research, with the aim of producing knowledge and practices about social occupational therapy, the populations and issues concerned, and the social role of occupational therapists.[8]

An example from Chile: Cintras is an organization that has worked across the country supporting victims of human rights violations such as torture, exile, political persecution, execution, or disappearance of family members since 1985 (Cintras, 2019). Occupational therapists work in interdisciplinary teams by recreating trusting social networks and life projects. A not-for-profit organization called EPES (for its acronym in Spanish: Educación Popular En Sud/Popular Health Education) looked at health promotion and education in human rights using an educational approach based on Freire's (1994) work (EPES, n.d.). This was a response to create community capacity and community leaders in health, education, and human rights. As part of EPES, occupational therapists had the opportunity to participate in the creation of sustainable educational material and initiatives in close collaboration with local communities in their territories in response to local demands (EPES, n.d.). Both practices were grounded in the idea of emancipatory practice (Freire, 1994), which goes beyond the biomedical model, making use of what they called a committed bond for all professionals working in the field of enabling dignifying social processes (Lira, Becker, & Castillo, 1989). This commitment was expressed through the explicit disclosure of the political position against neoliberalism and public participation in human-rights movements by healthcare professionals.

These two examples are examples of how intercultural translations (de Sousa Santos, 2014) can occur. In the case of Brazil and Chile, commonalities can be found in terms of how recent political instability pushed the profession (which was grounded in Global North ways of thinking and doing) to act (practice) and think (knowledge development) *socially*. The actual expression of these practices differs from country to country given local conditions of life, colonization, and history. It is essential to carefully consider how these new ways of understanding our professional ways of thinking and doing (coming from the South and in dialogue with the North) are expressed.

8 For theoretical issues and applied examples, please see Lopes and Malfitano (2021).

Vignette 4: From a Not-in-My-Backyard (NIMBY) Approach to Let's Open the Door and Welcome Some Help

Here we expand the expression "Not in My Backyard" (NIMBY), which brings to mind a person or a group (usually middle-class communities) who actively resist something happening. The *something* is needed (e.g., new infrastructure), but it is perceived as having potentially negative consequences for the residents. The expression has been used to describe those who engage in active resistance to new developments nearby where the person or groups live. Understanding the impact that social conditions, inequality, and politics have in anyone's occupations and our professional practice might be uncomfortable for the Global North. However, it is necessary for the Global North to understand what is happening in their backyards. Our claim here is that the benefits of embedding a social view as the norm in occupational therapy in the Global North will surpass the initial discomfort (which is common during building processes as in the NIMBY metaphor) and will bring the opportunity to tackle many of the common issues communities there are experiencing.

Intercultural translations: Going forward on the dialogues between the South and the North

Taff and Putnam (2022) make an open call to reflect on how *Northern* occupational therapy can be enacting and reproducing the neoliberal ways of thinking, doing, and learning worldwide. This is not a new concern. Hammell (2011) brought to the attention of the Global North the notion of theoretical imperialism within the profession. The prevalent focus of the profession on individual components (from skills to intrinsic motivation), disregarding complex economic, political, cultural, and legal circumstances, can be perceived as dangerous (Guajardo et al., 2015; Hammell, 2011). The idea of Global North and Global South as dichotomic epistemologies has been discussed by Meyers and Hunt (2014):

> [W]hen we speak of global health—this world of measurements, ambition, innovation, hierarchies, and sometimes venality—we would do well to remember it is not limited in practice or imaginations to formerly colonised worlds, from Africa to India, from post-Ottoman worlds to South America. Wherever extreme inequality, catastrophe, disaster, and war enter, those same zones may encounter and often come to rely on global health knowledge and practices. (p. 1922)

Recent changes in the geographical distribution of power and the dynamics between the Global South and Global North are reshaping how education, knowledge dissemination, and healthcare services (including occupational therapy) should be provided. Some of these changes include (but are not limited to) sociopolitical conflicts (revindication of Indigenous rights, wars, forced migration waves), changes in academic requirements for professional training (graduate competencies) either in national or regional levels, and the internationalization of scientific knowledge within the profession. In the experience of one of the co-authors in France, one of the turning points for changing education and practice in social occupational therapy was the experience of PRACTS (for its acronym in French: PRévention et promotion de la santé par des Activités Collectivisantes sur les TerritoireS/Prevention and health promotion through collective activities in the territories), which allows trainers to learn from the reality of the social occupational therapy practice and the social groups with different stakeholders. This is an initial experience, but more is required. We see this chapter as an opportunity for reflection, for opening dialogues between the Global North and South in the discipline, and for occupational therapy to embrace its call and social contract, by supporting all people to engage in what matters to them.

How Did We Experience Our Own Dialogues Between the South and the North?

Personal reflection (DC): An Australian occupational therapist came to me to say that once they were exposed to the Global South knowledges, "everything I once loved, it is now ruined" (personal communication). Their favorite children's books, cooking, and commercial films were now examined with a critical eye. The shows with European chefs "exploring" local cuisines in the Global South, once taken as an inspiration, were now seen as a living example of colonialism and disrespect for local cultures. The occupational therapist also described this experience as a "veil being lifted," as the idea of sociohistoric and political approaches in their professional training was absent in the early 2000s. After their initial "shock," they recognized that lifting the veil allowed them to see and understand the world in a richer and more complex way. We hope this chapter ruins things by lifting the veils for many occupational therapy students and practitioners in the Global North.

Personal reflection (MM): Epistemic violence—my own experience of the exotification of community-based approaches and inclusion of other knowledge when conducting my Ph.D. studies. Only empirical studies seem to be accepted as fulfilling legitimated forms to produce academic knowledge in a medical university in the Global North. My persistence in adopting a collaborative approach was framed as exotic, innovative, "ground-breaking" in my university, or aligning with emerging transformative frameworks within occupational science in the international community. I read this as epistemic violence, ignorance, and silencing other knowledges and traditions developed elsewhere and the strong presence of welfare systems that had prevented the application of community-based approaches as an urgent necessity.

Personal reflection (AM): In France, the notion of politics is frowned upon, and it is proclaimed in schools that the occupational therapist must be politically neutral. However, our remarks from the more social approaches are often considered as belonging to political and militant revindications, contrary to this principle of neutrality. When meeting novice occupational therapists in PRACTS as well as the students, they usually ask me how to reconcile a practice that considers political aspects without derogating from the rule of neutrality of a civil servant in the country. They assume that the only solution would be to work in a private or a nongovernmental organization as if public policies were not behind our professional practice. This is not unique to occupational therapists.

Personal reflection (LF): Exotifying the "social" not only places the diversity and richness of knowledges coming from the Global South into the margins but also makes it hard to put them in conversation with approaches from the North. I have been in conversations where the social is just "something" that you use when working with people in poverty or social exclusion, when enacting community-based approaches in practice, or when using participatory approaches in research. Then it is hard to dialogue regarding the social when trying to apply this thinking to privileged and unprivileged groups and to the implications in occupational therapy practice, education, and research. If the social is something that can be applied somewhere else, then it is very difficult to learn from the Global South and North.

Conclusion

We see this chapter as an opportunity for reflection, for exploring and revealing some of the ongoing dialogues between the Global North and South, and for occupational therapy to embrace its call and social contract, by supporting all people to engage in what matters to them. The idea of the social cannot be separated from the daily existences of local communities in the Global South. As a result, occupational therapy has evolved and developed practices to respond to the realities it is implementing. These realities are heavily influenced and determined by sociohistorical processes (such as dictatorships, economic models, and colonization) and determine people's doing in a situated manner.

Take-home message

In the words of Taff and Putnam (2022), we invite you as a reader to unmask, disentangle, and dismantle your own ways of doing and knowing in the profession if you are in the Global North. But we also ask those of you located in the Global South to carefully examine those taken-for-granted assumptions about life and human doing. And if you are one of us, someone who has moved across the world, be mindful of how the dialogues will appear as some clear (or not) possibilities in practice and knowledge development.

References

Barros, D. D., Ghirardi, I., & Lopes, R. E. (2002). Terapia ocupacional social. *Revista de Terapia Ocupacional da Universidade de Sao Paulo, 13*(3), 95–103. https://doi.org/10.11606/issn.2238-6149.v13i3p95-103

Beghin, N. (2022). Decoloniality as the only pathway to the right to development in Latin America. *Development, 65*(2–4), 178–185. https://doi.org/10.1057/s41301-022-00349-w

Bianchi, P. C., & Malfitano, A. P. S. (2022). Occupational therapy in Latin America: Conceptual discussions on territory and community. *Scandinavian Journal of Occupational Therapy, 29*(3), 210–218. https://doi.org/10.1080/11038128.2020.1842492

Bourdieu, P. (1993). *La Misère du monde.* Seuil.

Castel, R. (1995). *Les Métamorphoses de la Question Sociale.* Folio.

Castro, D., Dahlin-Ivanoff, S., & Mårtensson, L. (2014). Occupational therapy and culture: A literature review. *Scandinavian Journal of Occupational Therapy, 21*(6), 401–414. https://doi.org/10.3109/11038128.2014.898086

CEPAL – Comisión Económica para América Latina y el Caribe. (2022). *Panorama Social de America Latina y el Caribe: La Transformación de la Educación como Base para el Desarrollo Sustentable.* https://repositorio.cepal.org/server/api/core/bitstreams/15cfc3c4-9095-47c5-add6-c1b6205a3365/content

Cintras. (2019). Centro de Salud Mental y Derechos Humanos. Cintras. https://cintras.org/quienes.htm

Connell, R. (2007). *Southern Theory: The Global Dynamics of Knowledge in Social Science.* Allen & Unwin.

Correia, R. L., Wertheime, L. G., Morrison, R., & Silva, C. R. (2021). Contemporary perspectives of occupational therapy in Latin America: Contributions to the local dialogue. *South African Journal of Occupational Therapy, 51*(4), 41–50. https://doi.org/10.17159/2310-3833/2021/vol51n4a6

de Sousa Santos, B. (2007). *Cognitive Justice in a Global World: Prudent Knowledges for a Decent Life.* Lanham.

de Sousa Santos, B. (2014). *Epistemologies of the South: Justice Against Epistemicide.* Paradigm.

Dos Santos, V. (2017). Occupational therapy across South America: An overview of its backgrounds, current situation, and some contemporary issues. In D. Sakellariou & N. Pollard

(Eds.), *Occupational Therapies Without Borders: Integrating Justice with Practice* (2nd edn, pp. 203–210). Elsevier.

Duarte Cuervo, C., & Talero Cabrejo, P. (2022). Inequidades en la difusión y visibilidad del conocimiento: ¿Por qué deberían importarnos? *Revista Ocupación Humana, 22*(1), 3–11. https://doi.org/10.25214/25907816.1372

EPES. (n.d.). Fundación Educación Popular en Salud. EPES. https://epes.cl/quienes_somos/#resena

Farias, L. (2020). The (Mis)shaping of health: Problematizing neoliberal discourses of individualism and responsibility. In H. Hosseini, J. Goodman, S. C. Motta, & B. K. Gills (Eds.), *The Routledge Handbook of Transformative Global Studies* (pp. 268–281). Routledge.

Fassin, D. (2004). *Des Maux Indicibles: Sociologie des Lieux d'Écoute*. La Découverte.

Francisco, B. R. (1988). *Terapia Ocupacional*. Papirus.

Freire, P. (1994). *Pedagogy of Hope*. Continuum.

Galheigo, S. (2011). What needs to be done? Occupational therapy responsibilities and challenges regarding human rights. *Australian Occupational Therapy Journal, 58*(2), 60–66. https://doi.org/10.1111/j.1440-1630.2011.00922.x

Galheigo, S. M., Braga, C. P., Arthur, M. A., & Matsuo, C. M. (2018). Produção de conhecimento, perspectivas e referências teórico-práticas na terapia ocupacional brasileira: Marcos e tendências em uma linha do tempo. *Cadernos Brasileiros De Terapia Ocupacional, 26*(4), 723–738. https://doi.org/10.4322/2526-8910.ctoAO1773

Galvani, D., Barros, D. D., Pastore, M. D. N., & Sato, M. T. (2016). Exercícios etnográficos como atividades em espaço público: Terapia ocupacional social no fazer da arte, da cultura e da política. *Cadernos de Terapia Ocupacional da UFSCar, 24*(4), 859–868. https://doi.org/10.4322/0104-4931.ctoARF1004

Garzón López, P. (2013). Pueblos indígenas y decolonialidad: Sobre la colonización epistemológica occidental. *Andamios, 10*(22), 305–331. https://doi.org/10.29092/uacm.v10i22.278

Gonçalves, M. V., & Malfitano, A. P. S. (2020). Brazilian youth experiencing poverty: Everyday life in the favela. *Journal of Occupational Science, 27*(3), 311–326. https://doi.org/10.1080/14427591.2020.1757495

Granda, E. (2004). ¿A qué llamamos salud colectiva hoy? *Revista Cubana de Salud Pública, 30*(2). http://scielo.sld.cu/scielo.php?script=sci_arttext&pid=S0864-34662004000200009

Guajardo, A. (2016). Lecturas y relatos históricos de la terapia ocupacional en Suramérica: Una perspectiva de reflexión crítica. *Revista Ocupación Humana, 16*(2), 110–117. http://dx.doi.org/10.25214/25907816.141

Guajardo, A. (2020). About new forms of colonization in occupational therapy: Reflections on the idea of occupational justice from a critical-political philosophy perspective. *Cadernos Brasileiros de Terapia Ocupacional, 28*(4), 1365–1381. https://doi.org/10.4322/2526-8910.ctoARF2175

Guajardo, A., Kronenberg, F., & Ramugondo, E. (2015). Southern occupational therapies: Emerging identities, epistemologies and practices. *South African Journal of Occupational Therapy, 45*(1), 3–10.

Guajardo, A., & Mondaca, M. (2017). Human rights, occupational therapy and the centrality of social practices. In D. Sakellariou & N. Pollard (Eds.), *Occupational Therapies Without Borders: Integrating Justice with Practice* (2nd edn, pp. 102–108). Elsevier.

Hammell, K. W. (2011). Resisting theoretical imperialism in the disciplines of occupational science and occupational therapy. *British Journal of Occupational Therapy, 74*(1), 27–33. https://doi.org/10.4276/030802211X12947686093602

Hammell, K. W. (2021). Building back better: Imagining an occupational therapy for a post-COVID-19 world. *Australian Occupational Therapy Journal, 68*(5), 444–453. https://doi.org/10.1111/1440-1630.12760

Harvey, D. (2005). *A Brief History of Neoliberalism*. Oxford University Press.

Jansen van Vuuren, J., Okyere, C., & Aldersey, H. (2020). The role of occupational therapy in Africa: A scoping review. *South African Journal of Occupational Therapy, 50*(3), 3–21. https://dx.doi.org/10.17159/2310-3833/2020/vol50no3a2

Lees, N. (2021). The Brandt Line after forty years: The more North–South relations change, the more they stay the same? *Review of International Studies, 47*(1), 85–106. https://doi.org/10.1017/S026021052000039X

Lira, E., Becker, D., & Castillo, M. I. (1989). Psicoterapia de víctimas de represión política bajo dictadura: Un desafío terapéutico, teórico y político. In D. Becker and E. Lira (Eds.), *Derechos Humanos: Todo Es Según el Dolor con Que Se Mira* (pp. 17–41). Instituto Latinoamericano de Salud Mental y Derechos Humanos.

Lopes, R. E., & Malfitano, A. P. S. (2021). *Social Occupational Therapy: Theoretical and Practical Design*. Elsevier.

Loveman, B. (1986). Military dictatorship and political opposition in Chile, 1973–1986. *Journal of Interamerican Studies and World Affairs, 28*(4), 1–38. https://doi.org/10.2307/165745

Magalhães, L., Farias, L., Rivas-Quarneti, N., Alvarez, L., & Malfitano, A. P. S. (2019). The development of occupational science outside the Anglophone sphere: Enacting global collaboration. *Journal of Occupational Science, 26*(2), 181–192. https://doi.org/10.1080/14427591.2018.1530133

Maldonado-Torres, N. (2007). On the coloniality of being: Contributions to the development of a concept. *Cultural Studies, 21*(2), 240–270. https://doi.org/10.1080/09502380601162548

Malfitano, A. P. S. (2022). An anthropophagic proposition in occupational therapy knowledge: Driving our actions towards social life. *World Federation of Occupational Therapists Bulletin, 78*(2), 70–82. https://doi.org/10.1080/14473828.2022.2135065

Marques, A. (2010). *Construire Sa Légitimité au Quotidien: Le Travail Micropolitique autour d'une Équipe Mobile de Psychiatrie-Précarité*. École des Hautes Études en Sciences Sociales.

Marques, A. C. S., & Deranty, J.-P. (2017). La précarisation de la citoyenneté: Une étude comparative entre Brésil et France sur les difficultés de la construction d'une identité citoyenne pour les personnes en situation de précarité. In M. Bogalska Martin, D. Fernandez Varas, O. Leservoisier, & A. Martig (Eds.), *Itinéraires de Reconnaissance*. Editions des Archives Contemporaines.

Max-Neef, M. (2010). The need for an anti-neoliberal therapy. World Federation of Occupational Therapists (WFOT). https://archive.wfot.org/wfot2010/docs/Manfred_Max_Neef_ENG.pdf

Meyers, T., & Hunt, N. R. (2014). The other global South. *The Lancet, 384*(9958), 1921–1922. https://doi.org/10.1016/S0140-6736(14)62270-4

Mignolo, W. D. (2021). Coloniality and globalization: A decolonial take. *Globalizations, 18*(5), 720–737. https://doi.org/10.1080/14747731.2020.1842094

Nascimento, B. A. (1990). Contribuição à definição de uma política de extensão para o curso de T.O. da UFSCar. *Cadernos de Terapia Ocupacional da UFSCar, 1*(1), 7–12.

Occupational Therapy Professional Alliance of Canada. (2014). *Joint Position Statement: Diversity*. https://view.officeapps.live.com/op/view.aspx?src=https%3A%2F%2Fwww.acotup-acpue.ca%2FEnglish%2Fdocuments%2FJointPositionStatementonDiversityFINALrevision-25March2014.doc&wdOrigin=BROWSELINK

OECD. (2020). How's Life? 2020: Measuring Well-Being. www.oecd.org/wise/how-s-life-23089679.htm

Olivares-Aising, D. (2018). Occupational justice and human scale development: A theoretical integration approach. *Journal of Occupational Science, 25*(4), 474–485. https://doi.org/10.1080/14427591.2018.1513780

Owens, J., Singh, G., & Cribb, A. (2019). Austerity and professionalism: Being a good healthcare professional in bad conditions. *Health Care Analysis, 27*, 157–170. https://doi.org/10.1007/s10728-019-00372-y

Paugam, S. (1996). *L'Exclusion, l'État des Savoirs*. La Découverte.

Quijano, A. (2007). Coloniality and modernity/rationality. *Cultural Studies, 21*(2–3), 168–178. https://doi.org/10.1080/09502380601164353

Real Academia Española. (n.d). Social. In *Diccionario de la Lengua Española*. https://dle.rae.es/social?m=form

Rodríguez, J. P. (2021). The politics of neoliberalism in Latin America: Dynamics of resilience and contestation. *Sociology Compass, 15*(3), e12854. https://doi.org/10.1111/soc4.12854

Rotarou, E. S., & Sakellariou, D. (2017). Neoliberal reforms in health systems and the construction of long-lasting inequalities in health care: A case study from Chile. *Health Policy, 121*(5), 495–503. https://doi.org/10.1016/j.healthpol.2017.03.005

Taff, S. D., & Putnam, L. (2022). Northern philosophies and professional neocolonialism in occupational therapy: A historical review and critique. *Cadernos Brasileiros de Terapia Ocupacional, 30*, e2986. https://doi.org/10.1590/2526-8910.ctoAO22642986

Valderrama, C. (2019). Occupational therapies of the South: A proposal for its understanding. *Cadernos Brasileiros de Terapia Ocupacional, 27*(3), 671–680. https://doi.org/10.4322/2526-8910.ctoARF1859

Vidal, M. (1988). *El Hombre Inconcluso*. Colección Cintras.

Visvanathan, S. (1997). *A Carnival for Science: Essays on Science, Technology and Development*. Oxford University Press.

World Federation of Occupational Therapists. (2022). Occupational Therapy Human Resources Project 2022 – Numerical. WFOT. www.wfot.org/resources/occupational-therapy-human-resources-project-2022-numerical

Xypas, C., & Wallenhorst, N. (2020). La citoyenneté au défi des classes sociales au Brésil et en France. *Bildungsforschung, 1*(S), 1–21. https://doi.org/10.25656/01:19287

Yakushko, O. (2018). Witches, charlatans, and old wives: Critical perspectives on history of women's indigenous knowledge. *Women & Therapy, 41*(1–2), 18–29. https://doi.org/10.1080/02703149.2017.1323474

Zhang, Y., Andrew, J., & Rudkin, K. (2012). Accounting as an instrument of neoliberalisation? Exploring the adoption of fair value accounting in China. *Accounting, Auditing & Accountability Journal, 25*(8), 1266–1289. https://doi.org/10.1108/09513571211275470

Subject Index

Author Index